ENERGY EVERY DAY

Ron Woods
Chris Jordan
with the Human Performance Institute

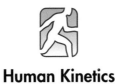

Human Kinetics

Library of Congress Cataloging-In-Publication Data

Woods, Ron, 1943 Nov. 6-
 Energy every day / Ron Woods, Chris Jordan ; with the Human
Performance Institute.
    p. cm.
 Includes bibliographical references and index.
 ISBN-13: 978-0-7360-8208-2 (soft cover)
 ISBN-10: 0-7360-8208-5 (soft cover)
 1. Exercise. 2. Physical fitness. 3. Health. 4. Fatigue.
I. Jordan, Chris, 1949- II. Title.
 RA781.W66 2010
 613.7--dc22
                              2009029106

ISBN-10: 0-7360-8208-5 (print)   ISBN-10: 0-7360-8612-9 (Adobe PDF)
ISBN-13: 978-0-7360-8208-2 (print)   ISBN-13: 978-0-7360-8612-7 (Adobe PDF)

Copyright © 2010 by Human Performance Institute

All rights reserved. Except for use in a review, the reproduction or utilization of this work in any form or by any electronic, mechanical, or other means, now known or hereafter invented, including xerography, photo-copying, and recording, and in any information storage and retrieval system, is forbidden without the written permission of the publisher.

This publication is written and published to provide accurate and authoritative information relevant to the subject matter presented. It is published and sold with the understanding that the author and publisher are not engaged in rendering legal, medical, or other professional services by reason of their authorship or publication of this work. If medical or other expert assistance is required, the services of a competent professional person should be sought.

Notice: Permission to reproduce the following material is granted to instructors and agencies who have purchased *Energy Every Day:* pp. 76 and 95, and Appendix 6 on p. 222. The reproduction of other parts of this book is expressly forbidden by the above copyright notice. Persons or agencies who have not purchased *Energy Every Day* may not reproduce any material.

The Web addresses cited in this text were current as of July 2009, unless otherwise noted.

Acquisitions Editor: Tom Heine; **Developmental Editor:** Mandy Eastin-Allen; **Assistant Editor:** Laura Pode-schi; **Copyeditor:** Tom Tiller; **Proofreader:** Leigh Keylock; **Permission Manager:** Martha Gullo; **Graphic Designer:** Fred Starbird; **Graphic Artist:** Kim McFarland; **Cover Designer:** Keith Blomberg; **Photographer (cover):** EyeWire; **Photographer (interior):** Neil Bernstein, unless otherwise noted; **Photo Asset Manager:** Laura Fitch; **Visual Production Assistant:** Joyce Brumfield; **Photo Production Manager:** Jason Allen; **Art Manager:** Kelly Hendren; **Associate Art Manager and Illustrator:** Alan L. Wilborn; **Printer:** United Graphics

Human Kinetics books are available at special discounts for bulk purchase. Special editions or book excerpts can also be created to specification. For details, contact the Special Sales Manager at Human Kinetics.

Printed in the United States of America   10   9   8   7   6   5   4   3   2   1

The paper in this book is certified under a sustainable forestry program.

Human Kinetics
Web site: www.HumanKinetics.com

United States: Human Kinetics
P.O. Box 5076
Champaign, IL 61825-5076
800-747-4457
e-mail: humank@hkusa.com

Canada: Human Kinetics
475 Devonshire Road Unit 100
Windsor, ON N8Y 2L5
800-465-7301 (in Canada only)
e-mail: info@hkcanada.com

Europe: Human Kinetics
107 Bradford Road
Stanningley
Leeds LS28 6AT, United Kingdom
+44 (0) 113 255 5665
e-mail: hk@hkeurope.com

Australia: Human Kinetics
57A Price Avenue
Lower Mitcham, South Australia 5062
08 8372 0999
e-mail: info@hkaustralia.com

New Zealand: Human Kinetics
Division of Sports Distributors NZ Ltd.
P.O. Box 300 226 Albany
North Shore City
Auckland
0064 9 448 1207
e-mail: info@humankinetics.co.nz

E4778

*To my wife, Kathy, who unfailingly supports
my passion to share my fascination and love of
physical activity and sports with the world.*

RBW

*To my parents, Maureen and David, for their
support and encouragement, and to Chanda
for her positive energy and spirit.*

CJ

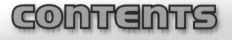

CONTENTS

PREFACE

If you've picked up this book, the chances are very good that you have struggled with a lack of personal energy. You are not alone. Most of us wish we had the time and energy to do more, experience more, achieve more, and spend more quality time with family and other loved ones.

In our role as performance coaches at the Human Performance Institute in Orlando, Florida, we have concluded that personal energy—not more time—is the key to leading a fulfilling life. Although we could all perhaps be better organized in our use of time, the fact remains that there is only so much time at our disposal. When it comes to energy, however, there is an unlimited supply within each of us, if only we know how to tap into it.

That's where this book comes in. We have based the book on the latest research from the sciences of nutrition, exercise physiology, and psychology as well as years of experience in training elite athletes and everyday people to improve their performance. This is not another diet or workout book; rather, it is a practical approach to using food for fuel and embracing enjoyable physical activities to give yourself more energy every day.

It seems clear to us that there must be a crisis of personal energy nowadays. We're bombarded with products that promise to deliver instant energy and a quick pick-me-up. Convenience stores advertise energy bars, energy drinks, and lots of other less-than-healthy snacks to give us a quick energy fix. Coffee shops count on their customers' need for a daily caffeine fix. And we still want more energy.

If you are looking for a permanent boost in your personal energy based on responsible science and practical application, then this book is for you. Not only will you feel more energetic; we guarantee that you'll perform better every day and become more fully engaged in life and with friends and family. These are powerful claims, but we feel confident in making them based on the results enjoyed by thousands of enthusiastic clients of the Human Performance Institute.

Our formula for success is pretty straightforward. You need to begin thinking about how you can create more personal energy and then manage it better. You will need to involve your mind, your body, your emotions, and even your spirit in order to get you where you want to go. But once you've unlocked the secrets to personal energy and made a personal habit of practicing them, you'll establish a lifestyle that sustains energy automatically.

Part I of this book lays the foundation for understanding the role that energy plays in your life. In chapter 1, you learn the importance of creating and maintaining a high level of energy in order to perform at your highest level and become fully engaged in your work and with friends and family. Understanding energy management involves accepting the role of each of the dimensions of your self—physical, emotional, mental, and spiritual—and how they interact with each other. We also help you see how critical the physical dimension is as the foundation of all our personal energy.

In chapter 2, we explore the sources of physical energy: nutrition, hydration, sleep, rest, movement, and breathing regulation. Chapter 3 provides a more thorough look at using food as the fuel for producing more energy by adopting strategies based on the latest science.

Chapter 4 leads you through a self-assessment to determine how ready you are for a change in lifestyle. We help you begin to understand the concept of self-motivation and how to channel it to your advantage. We also help you understand the value of stress for growth as well as how to cultivate a new attitude toward using stress to your advantage by making sure it is followed by rest and recovery.

Part II guides you through the process of gathering information about your current state, choosing a variety of new physical activities to explore, investigating their practicality, and developing a personal plan for physical activity.

Chapter 5 helps you assess your current level of physical fitness in order to establish a baseline and, over time, to measure improvement. Chapter 6 opens up a wide range of physical activities, including recreational sports and games, for you to consider based on your personal preferences, prior experiences, and needs. We encourage you to choose activities that are fun for you and that you will look forward to participating in regularly.

Once you've targeted a half dozen or so physical activities, chapter 7 asks you to gather more detailed information about those activities, then guides you through the key questions to consider for each one. Finally, chapter 8 assists you in laying out a personal, 2-week plan for physical activity that is tailored just for you and is practical to pursue. By this time, you should be excited, motivated, and eager to begin a new life phase through vigorous physical activity on a regular basis.

Part III helps you put your plan into action. Chapter 9 provides the nuts and bolts of how to make your plan work to produce high energy; specifically, it offers advice about breathing techniques, attitude adjustment, food, and hydration. Equally important, the chapter gives you instruction on the role of and techniques for warming up before activity and cooling down afterward; it includes specific exercises for improving flexibility and speeding up recovery. Finally, this chapter exposes you to various methods and equipment for strength training by listing pros and cons and showing demonstration photos of exercises for building muscular strength and endurance in key areas of the body.

Chapter 10 shows you how to keep a record of your progress as compared with the goals you set for yourself. You'll see the value of keeping an activity log and using a personal journal to record thoughts and feelings daily. After 6 or 8 weeks, you need to test yourself again to measure improvements and modify your activity plan based on the results. One of the keys to changing your behavior for the long term is to understand the role of daily rituals that become life habits after 90 days. These new habits form the foundation for a new lifestyle in which you produce more energy and use it more wisely.

In chapter 11, we lay out the typical barriers that people face in trying to make the changes we suggest. We think you will be glad to have a plethora of strategies to use in overcoming your barriers and will draw confidence from the knowledge that others have conquered their own barriers.

In chapter 12, we conclude with a quick review of the major concepts presented throughout the book in order to set them firmly in your mind. We encourage you to become your own personal coach in moving toward a high-energy lifestyle and to keep expanding your knowledge and understanding of the process. We also encourage you to build a strong network of supportive folks who will help you along the way by providing both emotional support and practical advice.

Our hope is that your journey toward a lifestyle of higher energy will help you achieve more success in every important area of your life. Even better, we think you should have *fun* along the way. Our aim is to help you see that generating more physical energy and managing it more effectively results in a healthier, more rewarding lifestyle that you can enjoy every day.

For more information on energy management, visit www.energyforperformance.com or make use of our educational offerings in person or by using the books and audio recordings available through our headquarters in Orlando.

ACKNOWLEDGMENTS

We are grateful to Rainer Martens, founder of Human Kinetics, who lent his support and artful guidance of this project during the initial germination of the idea and helped formulate the approach to the widest possible audience of folks who crave more energy today.

We also appreciate the early expert guidance of our acquisitions editor, Tom Heine, who enthusiastically supported this project, provided early feedback on the concept, chapter headings, and content, and helped focus the intended audience. Similarly, Mandy Eastin-Allen, who served as our developmental editor, lent her insightful analysis and practical advice throughout the writing and editing process with good humor and professionalism. Near the end of the project, Laura Podeschi smoothly assumed responsibility for shepherding us through the final days of revision and editing. Her ability to tie up loose ends with attention to detail along with her supportive spirit is much appreciated.

The founder of the Human Performance Institute, Dr. Jim Loehr, has been our enthusiastic supporter from the outset, and without his full pledge of cooperation and encouragement we could not have conceived this book. Much of the scientific and practical application of the broad concept presented in this book is the direct result of Jim's lifelong work to unravel the mysteries of maximizing personal energy and enable us to become fully engaged in every aspect of life.

Chris Osorio, President of Human Performance Institute, has been the voice of reason and practicality throughout the process but has been a zealous supporter of our efforts to promulgate the vision through this book to a wider audience. Jenn Lea and Stephanie Matos, as fitness coaches, helped us dig out valuable information and scientific verification and provided expert models for the stretching and strength training photos contained in chapter 9.

Finally, we are each grateful to the hundreds of clients of the Human Performance Institute who have shared their personal stories and struggles, solicited our help and guidance, and in the end became the inspiration for this book.

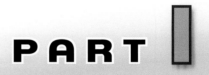

THE ENERGY SOLUTION

CHAPTER 1

BUILDING ENERGY FOR FULL ENGAGEMENT

In recent years, we've been bombarded by media reports on the world energy crisis due to the finite supply of raw materials from which our petroleum-based products are manufactured. Indeed, as worldwide demand for energy has risen, we've seen the dramatic effects of this crisis in our own lives. But most of us are also affected by another, equally insidious crisis—a *personal* energy crisis. For proof, simply glance at the plethora of energy-related products offered at any convenience store: energy bars, junk food, and lots of energy drinks. This apparent epidemic of low personal energy is likely to result in lower-quality performance at work, frustration in dealing with co-workers, and an inability to sustain high productivity over months and years.

After working long, hard hours that exceed the reliable capacity of the energy reserves we've accumulated, we find ourselves depleted and drained when we finally get home to family and friends. This cycle doesn't afford much opportunity to enjoy a good quality of life. Thus, for some of us, the cumulative stress of years of living without adequate personal energy not only causes poor work performance but also leads to damaged family relationships, poor health, unhappiness, and even depression.

Do you wish you had more energy for your spouse? Energy to play with your kids? Energy for activities for yourself? Better focus throughout the workday? Perhaps you have the time but lack the energy to fully interact with your spouse or family. After a long day, is it the best you can do to "zone out" in front of the television or play a computer game? Could you do better if you had more energy?

It's tempting to respond to depletion of energy reserves by trying a quick fix. Options include unhealthy junk food, sodas, energy drinks, energy bars, smoking, and pills. Sadly, each of these alternatives poses some risk to our health, and none really solves the problem. In fact, these quick fixes are likely to cause even more serious problems.

This chapter helps you understand that energy, rather than time, is your most precious resource. It is the energy you bring to the time you have that makes the difference. Desperately trying to find extra time in each day and rushing around to show up at as many commitments as you can does not lead to fulfilling, enjoyable, or productive moments. Rather, those times when you are full of energy and present in the moment have the most positive effect on your life. We want to help you become more aware of your current energy level and what you can do to keep your energy at a high level.

MORE ENERGY, NOT MORE TIME

We are often obsessed with time, and there never seems to be enough of it. We try to squeeze more into every minute of every day. We eat fast food on the run and chat on our cell phone while driving, eating, or exercising. At the end of the day, we fall into bed exhausted, but sleep doesn't come easily because we're worried about the next day.

In the business world, corporate trainers have seized on the concept of time management to help us organize and prioritize our time better in order to achieve more in less time. To be sure, such programs can be helpful; we can use them to stay better focused and make effective judgments about daily priorities. They are limited, however, by the fact that time itself is a finite resource. There are only 24 hours in each day (one-third of which are spent asleep). Thus, once we've planned our waking hours, we've reached our limit. Our PDAs (personal digital assistants) and laptops can list things to do, but they can't carry them out. We may have a plan for tasks to complete but little idea of how to use our time for efficient, productive functioning. Even when we're super-organized, it's not always possible to operate with purpose and high energy all day long.

Here's where personal energy management comes in. We propose to help you do two things: *produce more healthy natural energy and manage it more effectively.* Throughout this book, we help you understand how to create more personal energy by focusing on the physical side of energy creation. We show you how to optimize your physical energy and integrate it with your emotional, mental, and spiritual energy.

We also want your personal energy to be both renewable and sustainable. Learning how to renew your energy on a regular basis will rejuvenate and invigorate you and promote good health and appearance. Sustaining energy is a matter of adjusting your lifestyle so that your personal energy resources never become totally depleted or permanently damaged.

Consider the effect of high and low energy levels on your emotions. In figure 1.1, you can see four different cells that represent energy states as high or low and as either positive or negative. Typical feelings involving high positive energy are hopefulness, passion, challenge, and connection; other feelings of high positive energy are alertness, focus, enthusiasm, and optimistic attitude. This energy state gives you the opportunity to embrace challenges and respond

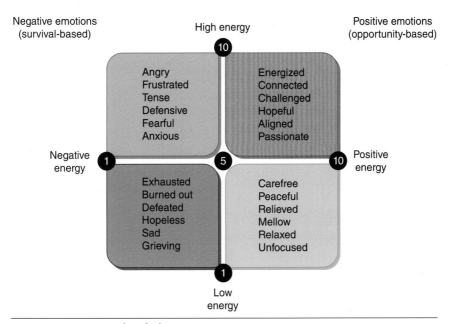

Figure 1.1   Energy level chart.

in a high-quality way. It is the only type of energy that fosters full engagement with life in the moment and therefore high performance.

Of course, you can also have high energy that is negative, and it carries with it the emotions of frustration, anger, anxiety, tenseness, and fear. While these feelings may spark a high level of energy, they also interfere with your thinking and decision making. They may be helpful in case of a physical emergency when your goal is simply to survive, but in most situations a high level of negative energy is counterproductive.

Sometimes you should intentionally experience *low* positive energy by strategically disengaging in order to allow yourself to rest and recover in your physical, emotional, mental, and spiritual dimensions. It is critical to spend sufficient time at this energy level in order to renew yourself and enable your embracing of the next challenge.

Low *negative* energy, on the other hand, leaves us feeling exhausted, burned out, sad, or hopeless. It can also be manifested in moodiness, irritability, and impatience. This category of energy may constitute a type of enforced recovery from stress and overwhelming challenge. It is critical that you develop skills to move out of this toxic level of negative energy.

In figure 1.1, energy level is represented on a scale of 1 (lowest) to 10 (highest). Negative or positive quality is also rated from 1 (lowest negative) to 10 (highest positive).

Unfortunately, after age 30 the demands on our energy typically continue to increase even as nature plays an evil trick on us by decreasing our natural energy capacity. Figure 1.2 shows the dramatic drop (green line) in energy after age 30.

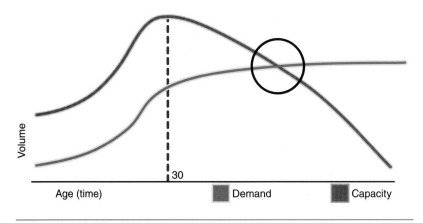

Figure 1.2   Demand versus capacity.

At the same time, our energy demands (red line) tend to peak in our 40s and 50s in the form of work responsibilities, family involvements, and other obligations.

It's pretty clear, then, that the years ahead will be challenging unless you take steps now to minimize the natural energy loss that is coming your way. Our goal is to help you manage your physical energy through methods that allow you to function at a high level of energy, deal effectively with pressure and stress, and overcome the sense of time shortage. Along the way, we highlight the importance of built-in recovery time to help you recharge, refresh, and face a new day.

MORE ENERGY FOR FULL ENGAGEMENT

We believe that producing and managing more personal energy allows you to live a more engaged life. When your energy level is high, it allows you to become fully engaged in the life activities that really matter to you. High energy drives the engagement process, whereas a lack of energy undermines it. What exactly is full engagement?

Full engagement is an acquired skill that enables you to invest your full and best energy—right here, right now.

This definition's key implication is that the capacity for full engagement can be developed. That's good news. It means that you are not locked out by heredity, environment, or age. You can learn to live your life in full engagement with meaningful work, relationships, and causes.

A second characteristic of full engagement is that we must focus our full energy and attention on the present rather than on the past or the future. Only by fully committing ourselves to being present-centered can we hope to maximize our effort and deliver our best possible performance. This does not mean that we should fail to learn life lessons from the past, nor that we should never plan or think about the future. It does mean that you will benefit from investing your best energy in the here and now. Even if your current task involves planning for the future, you are still doing so by expending energy in the present.

To feel the power of full engagement, have a conversation with a friend or business associate and focus your attention fully on that person for 1 minute. Ask a question and then actively listen to the response; to show interest, use body language such as strong eye contact and positive head nods. Focus your mind on the content of the answer as well as on the feeling your friend or associate conveys. In order to be sure you got it right, react to his or her answer with a question that summarizes your understanding of the answer. At the end of the minute, take stock of your skill and performance in active listening for full engagement. Is this a familiar pattern for you? Did you find it to be natural? Or was it difficult to achieve? Was your mind focused on the response, or were you thinking ahead to your next question? Did your body language convey interest, attention, and appropriate feeling?

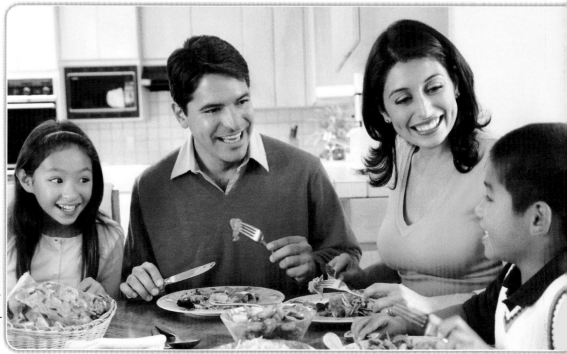

iStockphoto/Catherine Yeulet

Sharing a meal, these family members are fully engaged with each other.

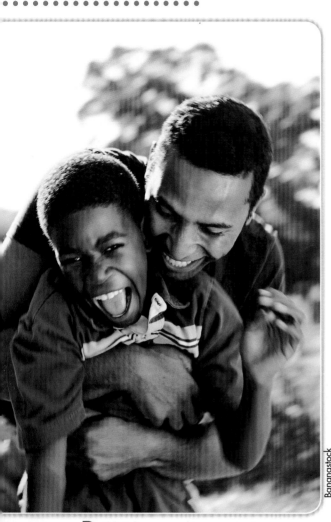

Daddy's home . . . time to play!

Are you able to deploy the mindset of full engagement throughout your daily life? Do you consistently engage fully with those around you, whether they be associates at work or family or friends at home? If you have young children, here's a test of your ability to fully engage with them each day. If you arrive home from work to the sound of a child's voice squealing "[Daddy or Mommy] is home!" what's your next move? Is it to spend time giving full attention to your child or children? Do you touch them, listen to them, question them, hold them, play with them, and give them your undivided attention? The younger they are, the more limited their concept of time is—and the more crucial the immediacy of your attention to them.

Maybe you've gotten into the habit of saying a quick hello, then slipping away to change clothes, check your messages, look through the day's mail, or just sit down and relax. Can't those activities wait until later—after you spend time with loved ones? Sure, you need to unwind, relax, and decompress from a day at work; but if you say that family is a priority, perhaps you should embrace the opportunity to spend 15 minutes with those who are most important to you. If you simply lack the energy to interact, read on to find the secrets to expanding your energy capacity.

DIMENSIONS OF FULL ENGAGEMENT

Full engagement is characterized by balance among our physical, emotional, mental, and spiritual dimensions (see figure 1.3). The spiritual dimension referred to describes the depth, clarity, and intensity of the purpose and meaning in your life. It implies that we all have a clear vision and purpose for life and are fully committed and exhibit passion toward achieving that purpose. In addition, our actions are principle-centered and ethical in all aspects of life.

Frequently Asked Questions

Q: How can I unwind before I get home so that I am ready to engage my kids and spouse?

A: If you can swing it, stop by the gym on the way home or take a brief walk and let the physical activity help you recharge. Another good option is to play your favorite music during the drive home and practice some deep breathing exercises on the way. When you pull into the driveway, leave your cell phone or other electronic device in the car to remove all temptation to reconnect with work. You can retrieve them later if necessary—after your kids are busy doing homework or in bed.

Full engagement means living a life that is

- spiritually aligned with our purpose in life,
- mentally focused on the present moment,
- emotionally connected by positive energy, and
- physically energized.

The alternative means living a life that is

- lacking in purpose (nothing really matters),
- unfocused and scattered in thought,
- dominated by negative emotions (e.g., anger, fear, moodiness, irritability), and
- marked by constant fatigue and a feeling of being drained.

You may notice that the foundation of the pyramid shown in figure 1.3 is the *physical* side of our being. Living with low physical energy dramatically weakens our capacity to develop our emotional, mental, and spiritual skills. At our core, we are physical beings, and we have the capacity to develop our other dimensions only if we nurture and strengthen our physical side first.

Our research at the Human Performance Institute shows that of more than 12,000 clients surveyed, only 4 percent described themselves as "fully engaged" in a balanced, positive state

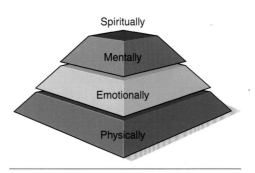

Figure 1.3 Pyramid of four dimensions.

of physical, emotional, mental, and spiritual energy. Compare that small percentage with the 51 percent who described themselves as "disengaged" (and another 3 percent who said they were "toxically disengaged"). If you're keeping score, this means that more than half of our clients place themselves on the negative side of the ledger and come to us looking for answers. And even among our clients who see themselves as "engaged" (about 42 percent), half admit to being physically disengaged. These alarming percentages are supported by an inarguable body of research knowledge that makes clear the following reality:

Physical energy is the foundation of all our energy—emotional, mental, and spiritual.

Physical fatigue, in contrast, compromises engagement; that is, it undercuts your ability to be positive, focused, productive, and passionate. Notice the computer worker's clear lack of energy below. Do you ever look or feel like that during a day?

CREATING PHYSICAL ENERGY

Physical energy comes from the interaction of oxygen and glucose in the cells of the body. Thus eating and breathing are the key systems for us to regulate in order to maximize our production of energy. Throughout this book, we discuss how you can create more physical energy by practicing smart nutrition and engaging in fun physical activities that improve your ability to fuel your body.

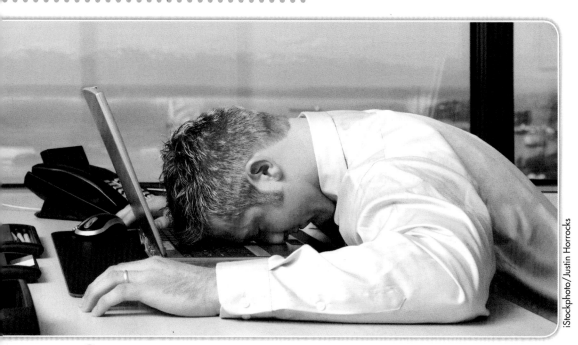

iStockphoto/Justin Horrocks

Got energy?

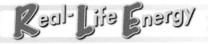

Real-Life Energy

When I attended the Corporate Athlete Course at the Human Performance Institute in 2007, I discovered that I was diabetic, had high blood pressure, and was in danger of having a stroke or heart attack. I began to realize that I was doing all the things that could shorten my life. I was eating the wrong way, I was always tired, and I didn't have time for my family or friends.

The course helped me learn how to develop daily rituals which, if used properly, can help enhance the quality of our lives. It also taught me how to develop mentally, physically, emotionally, and spiritually. I learned that a positive outlook on life can result from forming positive rituals.

Since then, I have lost more than 60 pounds (27 kilograms). I am energetic and have been able to handle situations effectively while avoiding getting too emotional. I have also felt enriched spiritually. I do not have the words to explain how much these changes have meant to me. The energy management concepts that I found most helpful in my journey to reach my ultimate mission in life are these: develop rituals, exercise regularly, and make time for recovery.

—*Betty Smith, housekeeping manager, The Breakers Palm Beach*

The food you eat gives you the fuel that keeps you alive and functioning. We explore this process in greater detail in chapter 3, which considers the essential role of glucose in the body and addresses other nutrients critical to optimal physical functioning. Water, of course, is also crucial, and though many of us know the importance of drinking enough water, we haven't necessarily developed the habit of consuming the recommended 8 to 10 cups (1.9 to 2.4 liters) each day. Yet learning to manage both your food and your fluid intake on a daily basis is essential for maximizing your physical energy. We suggest clear guidelines and practical tips for creating positive rituals and habits to ensure that you take in the basic fuel needed for your body to function well.

Most of us take breathing for granted; it's just something that comes naturally. But when we can't get enough oxygen because we're drowning, choking, or feeling panic, we suddenly become aware of breathing as a precious process. In fact, conscious regulation of our breathing can help us handle panic, fear, anxiety, anger, and pressure to perform. Deep abdominal breathing—rather than shallow breathing from the chest—changes our body chemistry, mood, level of relaxation, and ability to focus. Maintaining a fit, strong body with optimal posture enhances proper breathing and ensures more efficient delivery of oxygen to our cells. (For more in-depth discussion of deep breathing techniques, see chapter 9.)

Sleep is another critical factor in building your physical energy. We know that most of us require 7 to 8 hours of sleep each night, but few of us seem able to achieve that goal. Yet the mere routine of going to bed and waking up at consistent times every day helps improve the quality of sleep and maximizes our chance of waking up refreshed, rejuvenated, and eager to begin the day. Maintaining a consistent sleep pattern allows you to go into the typical stages of deep sleep that are necessary in order for your body to recharge. Sleep–wake cycles are based on the circadian rhythm of life and are hardwired into the biology of humans and other animals. Keeping to a regular sleep pattern helps you avoid sleep debt, which can be both uncomfortable and counterproductive. These habits can be learned and reinforced for all but a few of us; you might even want to try learning to nap properly during the day (see chapter 11 for more discussion of sleep strategies).

The beauty of sleep is that it allows us to recover from the energy demands and stresses of the day. But sleep isn't the only solution. We can learn to include recovery time throughout the day by changing our routine, taking breaks, and moving about. The key is to consciously acknowledge the need for recovery time and schedule it no matter what our task or activity.

The final piece of the puzzle in creating physical energy involves engaging in physical activity. It may seem counterintuitive to think that if you have little or no energy, you should exercise to acquire it. How is this possible? But the research is astounding, and physical activity does in fact help create and sustain a high level of energy. If you have recently been physically active, think back to how you felt immediately afterward. Did you feel energized, revved up, and ready for more? This is usually the case, unless you overdid the activity. In chapter 8, we help you develop your personal prescription for physical activity.

CREATING YOUR PERSONAL PLAN FOR PHYSICAL ACTIVITY

One of our key goals for this book is to help you develop and implement a custom-made plan for your physical activity. The evidence is clear-cut that just by moving your body you can develop a higher level of personal energy that permeates every facet of your life. Your simple challenge is to *create more physical energy, then manage it better.*

Most personal fitness books urge you to increase physical movement by taking up activities such as walking or stair climbing or by maximizing activity while doing household chores. Other books send you straight to a fitness center and prescribe daunting workouts with exercise machines and weight training equipment that often seem torturous in their boring, repetitive movements. Those seeking an easy way out are targeted by ubiquitous ads for exercise machines and routines that promise effective workouts in just minutes a day; they seem too good to be true, and they certainly are.

We propose instead that you expand your choices for physical activity to include a wide range of enjoyable pursuits that include recreational and competitive sport. We know from multiple research projects that some of us choose physical activities that relieve stress and help us relax. Others enjoy testing their sports skills under the pressure of competition. Some people enjoy just being outdoors while appreciating their natural surroundings. And perhaps a majority of us enjoy the social side of physical activity that allows us to build and nurture friendships. In fact, an increasing number of people of all ages have found that being physically active together with family members promotes family fun and strengthens relationships.

Whatever your motivation for physical activity, we want to help you get moving in ways that exhilarate you! Fun should be your objective, but smart planning increases the odds of having a good time—and repeating the quest for fun on a regular basis.

Let's get you started on a journey toward a higher level of physical energy through movement, physical activity, and sport. We guarantee that you'll set the stage for a life that is energized, healthier, and happier. (Note: Daily physical movements can be energizing, but physical activities connote a conscious effort to be physically active in play, walking, jogging, etc. Both are different from sports, which are organized, follow rules, and are generally competitive.)

TIPS for High Energy

- The key to performing better in all areas of your life is to focus not on carving out more time but on developing a higher level of energy.
- Developing a higher level of personal energy enables you to live a life characterized by full engagement.
- Full engagement involves balancing the four dimensions of your self—physical, emotional, mental, and spiritual.
- Physical energy is the foundation of all of our energy. It is the fundamental source of our capacity for full engagement that comes from the interaction of oxygen, glucose, and physical activity. It is also supported by adequate levels of water, sleep, and recovery time.
- To increase your personal energy level, you need to fashion a personal plan to create more energy and manage your energy better.

CHAPTER 2

UNLEASHING THE POWER OF PHYSICAL ENERGY

The sedentary work life that is reality for many of us today has led to an alarming reduction in physical activity. When we spend most of our time—and get paid for—using our minds rather than our bodies, we can fall into the trap of believing that the physical self is less important than the mental self. In fact, nothing could be further from the truth. Without physical energy as the foundation, our emotional, mental, and spiritual energy has no chance to flourish. Living without physical activity causes us to be less healthy and productive than we might be, and it dooms us to rapid decline as we age.

Let's quickly review the essential elements of producing physical energy:

- Movement
- Rest
- Nutrition
- Hydration
- Sleep (Note: Rest is relief or break from work or exertion or a change of activity. Sleep is one example of rest.)
- Breath regulation

Later chapters focus on nutrition, hydration, rest, sleep, and breath regulation. This chapter explains the critical importance of physical activity to our well-being. For many of us, physical activity can be the most difficult support to establish for our physical being. The challenge for many people is that physical activity in today's world is almost purely voluntary. Meeting this challenge requires you to acknowledge physical activity's purpose and importance and muster the enthusiasm and commitment to establish a routine of daily physical activity as part of your lifestyle. Whereas we simply must breathe and eat to live even a short while, we can exist for a long time without substantial physical movement. Yet to live without purposeful physical activity is to risk our health, our happiness, and life itself. This chapter looks at the evidence supporting this bold statement.

BENEFITS OF
REGULAR PHYSICAL ACTIVITY

Human beings were designed to move, to be physically active. Much of our body mass consists of muscle, which plays the role of literally pulling on our bony levers to make us move. As soon as we begin to move, a cascade of physiological and chemical events occurs to generate the energy needed to contract the muscles and move the body. Heart rate, body temperature, and metabolism all increase as hormones are released, fat is broken down, and glucose is sent to the muscles. This is all good news for our energy level, our health, and our feeling of well-being. Now, let's take a look at the specific benefits of physical activity to your physical, emotional, mental, and spiritual states.

Physical Benefits

 • Physical activity enhances your body's ability to use insulin, which regulates blood sugar, and maintain normal optimal blood sugar levels. This is a significant factor in light of the fact that one in four Americans is at risk for developing type 2 diabetes. Remember as well that glucose is one of the two foundations for your personal energy (The President's Council 1998).

 • Physical activity helps lower blood pressure, blood triglyceride level, and low-density lipoprotein (LDL, the "bad" cholesterol) and helps raise high-density lipoprotein (HDL, the "good" cholesterol), thus reducing the risk of heart disease, heart attack, and stroke, which, taken together, constitute the number one killer today in the United States. People who do not exercise regularly are twice as likely to develop heart disease as those who do (The President's Council 1998).

 • Physical activity may reduce the incidence of certain types of cancer, including cancers of the colon, breast, and female reproductive organs (National Cancer Institute 2008).

 • Physical activity enhances your appearance by positively altering your body composition—specifically, the proportion of fat to lean (muscle) tissue. Physical activity generally helps you lose fat mass while maintaining or even increasing lean mass.

 • Physical activity reduces the risk of being overweight or obese. Since overweight and obesity have reached epidemic proportions in the United States, more health professionals are touting the importance of nutrition and exercise in reducing body fat. Approximately two-thirds of Americans are overweight, and half of those are classified as obese. These statistics are based on body mass index (BMI), which is expressed as a ratio of body weight to height. Adults are generally considered overweight with a BMI of 25 to 29.9 and obese with a BMI of 30 or greater (National Center for Health Statistics 2004).

 • Physical activity slows aging and helps maintain a high quality of life even in later years. In fact, a physically active 60-year-old can achieve the same fitness level as an inactive 40-year-old, and that 20-year differential becomes pretty attractive as we hit "the big five-oh" (American College of Sports Medicine 2003).

Emotional Benefits

- Physical activity can make you feel more energetic, more self-confident, and just happier. It causes your body to produce chemicals called endorphins, which act as a kind of natural morphine and thus reduce pain and increase feelings of well-being; in fact, endorphins are responsible for the euphoric feeling called the "runner's high." Since endorphins decrease feelings of stress, physical activity can also alleviate symptoms of depression. Muscles tend to relax after physical activity, and a feeling of calm and satisfaction reduces tension in your body. Thus physical activity is a natural tranquilizer!

- During physical activity, neurotransmitters such as serotonin, norepinephrine, and dopamine reach elevated levels in the brain and have a powerful effect by regulating brain functions.

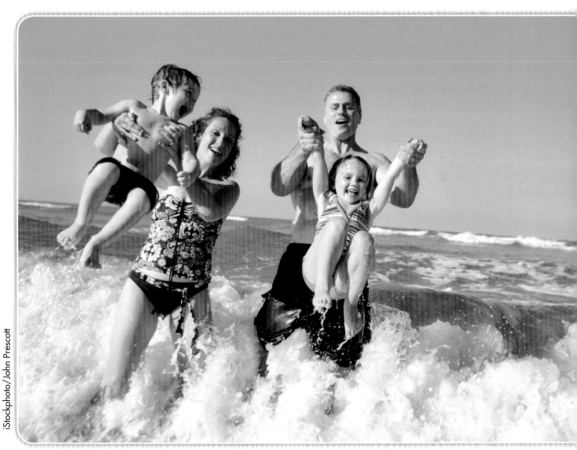

iStockphoto/John Prescott

A natural high through family physical activity.

- Body image tends to improve as your body shape and appearance become more attractive. Clothes fit better, and you draw admiring glances from friends and strangers. What an ego boost!
- You may also enjoy a sense of accomplishment if you engage in physical activity that enables you to gain mastery of a new sport or physical skill—or improve your performance in an old skill.

Mental Benefits

- The revolutionary discovery of neuroplasticity in recent years has opened up a vast new world of hopefulness even as we age. We used to think that the brain we were born with had a finite number of cells and that over time those cells gradually died without being replaced. Now, however, we have scientific evidence that our brain can grow and change at any age (Doidge 2007).
- Exercise can make you smarter! Recent research with middle and high school students in Naperville, Illinois, and Titusville, Pennsylvania, showed clearly that performing aerobic exercise early in the day improved focus, concentration, and retention of learning. In fact, when their performance on standardized tests was compared with 250,000 students from 38 countries around the world, the Naperville students ranked first in science and sixth in math.

  While Naperville spends a notably lower amount per pupil than other top-tier Illinois public schools, the school district consistently ranks among the top 10 in the state. In contrast, Titusville, Pennsylvania, is a nearly defunct small town of 6,000 residents where median income is $25,000 and 75 percent of kindergartners receive government assistance for school lunches. Scores on standardized tests by students at Titusville have risen from below the state average to 17 percent above it in reading and 18 percent above it in math (Ratey 2008).
- Exercise stimulates growth in your brain at any age. It clearly helps produce the number of nerve and brain cells from stem cells in your hippocampus. Much research has centered on the benefits of aerobic exercise, such as walking, jogging, swimming, and bicycling; these activities seem to stimulate creation of new brain cells if done regularly with at least a moderate level of exertion.
- Physical activity that requires decision making and tactical adjustments can strengthen and expand the neural networks in the brain. Thus, working on skill acquisition in any sport or activity is just as important to the brain as aerobic activity is to the body.
- The best way to enhance your brain through physical activity is to choose a sport or activity that challenges both the cardiovascular system and the brain. Good choices include tennis, dance, martial arts, Pilates, and yoga (Ratey 2008).

Spiritual Benefits

- Spiritual energy provides the depth, clarity, and intensity of the purpose and meaning in your life. This spiritual energy ensures that you can be fully

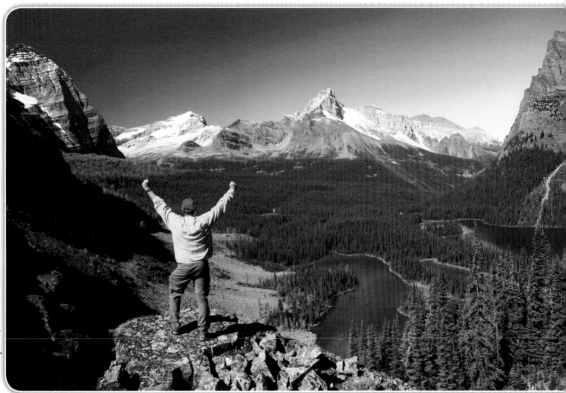

iStockphoto/Andrew Penner

Physical activity can have a spiritual side, too.

committed to your purpose in life and exhibit passion and enthusiasm toward your goals while never compromising your principles.

• Physical energy allows us to strive, achieve, and commit to our spiritual values. When we are short on physical energy, we become preoccupied with securing it and thus lose focus, waver in our commitments, and thrust our higher values to the background. Lack of energy can erode your passion, persistence, commitment, will to succeed, and ability to overcome life's relentless storms or challenges.

• Physical movement is the most powerful stimulant we know to overcome a lack of energy. Movement gets your blood flowing, raises metabolism, improves your mood, and sharpens your focus. All of these changes allow you to reach higher in order to meet the most critical spiritual challenges in your life (Loehr 2007).

We've shown you how physical activity affects every part of your being. If you have tended previously to see physical activity only in relation to its obvious physical benefits, we hope you now see a broader picture that includes your emotional, mental, and spiritual dimensions.

UNLEASHING YOUR PHYSICAL POWER

Let's take a look at the rituals and habits that are critical to maximizing your physical energy. Check the ones that you have already put in place, then circle those you still need to establish.

- ☐ Eat three meals and two snacks daily.
- ☐ Eat breakfast every day.
- ☐ Eat a balanced, healthy diet.
- ☐ Regulate portion sizes by using the guideline of five handfuls (use the size of your palm, not including fingers, to measure a handful).
- ☐ Never go longer than 4 hours without food.
- ☐ Drink water regularly throughout the day.
- ☐ Consume no more than two servings of alcohol per day. (Note: One serving equals 12 oz. of beer, 5 oz. of wine, or 1.5 oz. of liquor.)
- ☐ If you consume alcohol, do so with meals only.
- ☐ Consistently go to bed and get up at the same time.
- ☐ Get up early and go to bed early.
- ☐ Get up and move around or stretch every 90 minutes throughout the day.
- ☐ Engage in some type of physical activity every day.
- ☐ Complete at least two cardiorespiratory interval workouts each week.
- ☐ Do strength training at least twice a week.

Now that you have tallied your responses to the checklist, give yourself a pat on the back for the habits you have already established. Each one is helping you produce physical energy, and with the addition of a few others you'll start to see a dramatic difference. Now it's time to figure out how to add these new behaviors to your life. Our advice is to use the following principles.

Start by making the changes that are easiest for you. This may mean drinking more fluids, regulating sleep, or reducing meal portions. Each simple change you make reinforces your commitment, builds your confidence, and produces an immediate result. Once you've made these changes, stick with them for at least 60 days to make them permanent. Along the way, reward yourself at weekly intervals to celebrate your success; you might, for example, treat yourself to a massage, see a play or movie, or buy some new sports clothing.

Accept the fact that, because of your existing habits, some changes will be easier than others for you to make. For instance, if you were taught not to snack between meals, you may find it psychologically difficult to change that habit. After reading chapter 3, however, you'll realize how critical snacking is to the process of energy production; in fact, when it is combined with portion control at the three main meals, it works remarkably well. This is a case where two recommended habits complement each other and should be implemented at the same time. In fact, a third habit—drinking fluids throughout the day—fits nicely with the first two, since drinking more water reduces your perceived hunger.

One choice you have to make in order to pump up your physical energy is to engage in physical movement. Depending on your attitude toward and experience with physical activity, you might approach change in this area in any of multiple ways. For people who have heretofore included little unnecessary movement in daily life, it makes sense to start by incorporating stretching and large-muscle movements at 90-minute intervals throughout the day and perhaps adding a daily walk. You can invite your dog along, or not!

If you played a sport at some point in the past, think about how to get involved in it again, but remember to ease back into it. Ask yourself if it is affordable, convenient, fun, and appropriate for your age and fitness level; you may find that a favorite sport needs to be adjusted out of respect for your current age or ability. Before you return to a sport, it is helpful to do some general body conditioning in order to prepare for the increased demands of sporting activity. When you begin to play the sport again, limit the length and intensity

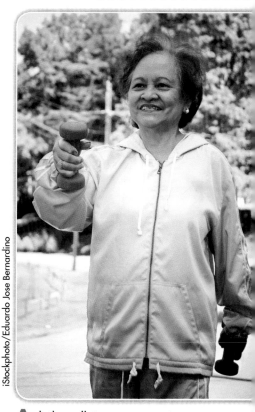

iStockphoto/Eduardo Jose Bernardino

A daily walk is a great routine at any age.

Frequently Asked Questions

Q: I used to play basketball in high school and have always loved the game. How would I go about getting back into the sport now that I am 45 and haven't been very active for more than 15 years?

A: After doing some general body conditioning by walking, running, and sprinting (with appropriate warm-up and cool-down rituals), ease back onto the court by shooting baskets and practicing your passing, dribbling, and defending skills. Next, play in small-sided games such as two-on-two and three-on-three. You might also consider joining a group of players who are close to you in age and size in order to minimize the chance of sustaining an injury or overextending yourself. If you eventually want to compete in a recreational basketball league, give yourself the best opportunity for fair competition by choosing one that is separated into divisions based on age.

of your play, then gradually build up to a level that is comfortable for you. The worst decision you can make is to launch an overly intense return that produces an injury and sets you back for weeks or even longer.

The rest of this book coaches you through many other questions about establishing a healthy program of physical activity that is fun, rewarding, and guaranteed to give you more physical energy.

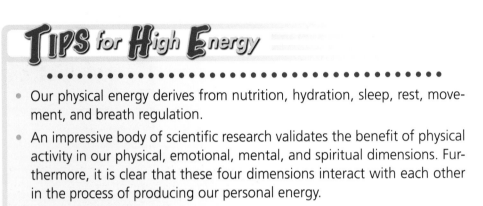

TIPS for High Energy

- Our physical energy derives from nutrition, hydration, sleep, rest, movement, and breath regulation.

- An impressive body of scientific research validates the benefit of physical activity in our physical, emotional, mental, and spiritual dimensions. Furthermore, it is clear that these four dimensions interact with each other in the process of producing our personal energy.

- Use the checklist of habits and rituals to assess your current behavior and begin to plan which new behaviors you need to add.

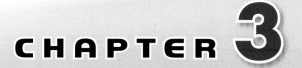

CHAPTER 3

ADDING HIGH-OCTANE FUEL

A book about personal energy must include a chapter on nutrition. It has to be discussed because food is our fuel for generating energy. That's right: *Food is fuel!* And without a steady supply of fuel, our bodies cannot produce energy efficiently. Although our focus in this book is on using physical activity to boost your energy, you need to make sure you are eating right in order to provide sufficient fuel for the process.

The purpose of this chapter is not to overwhelm you with details about the complex subject of nutritional science, but to provide you with simple guidelines for what to eat, when to eat, and how much to eat in order to manage and maximize your energy. We also provide a basic understanding of why it is so important to follow these guidelines correctly.

NEED VERSUS WANT

Let's start at the most basic level. Food is fuel, but it should also provide essential nutrients so that the body can function optimally. We need an optimally functioning body in order to manage and maximize our energy. Thus we must consider the nutrients we get (or don't get) from the food we consume.

We can divide the food we eat into two simple categories: "need" foods and "want" foods. Need foods, which are richer in nutrients and lower in calories, include grains, fruits, vegetables, low-fat dairy products, and lean meats. Want foods, which are lower in nutrients and higher in calories, include sweets, chips, fries, high-fat meats, soda, and alcohol.

It is important to discuss both need and want foods, both because eating should be a satisfying and enjoyable experience and because, in reality, eating well may involve consuming some of your favorite want foods! More important, any nutrition plan that prohibits ever eating your favorite want food is doomed to failure. That's why diets don't work in the long term. A more

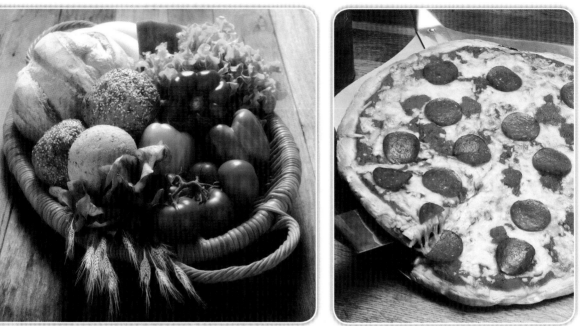

© Corbis (left); Zol—Fotolia.com (right)

The difference between "need" and "want" foods.

realistic, sustainable approach is *not* to eliminate any particular foods, but to manage what, when, and how much you eat.

So, is it possible to enjoy want foods and still manage your energy effectively? Absolutely! The keys are balance and portion control. We recommend a ratio of four to one—that is, four portions of need food to one portion of want food. This approach allows you to indulge a little yet control your energy. It probably sounds like a balance you can live with (it may even seem a bit generous), and that's the point. It *has* to be something you can live with for the rest of your life; otherwise, it will end up as nothing but another broken New Year's resolution.

EATING LIGHT AND OFTEN

The key to maintaining high energy is to eat light and often. If you think about this for a moment, it makes good sense. How do you feel after eating too much—after a large meal at the end of a long day, or after Thanksgiving dinner? Like most people, you probably feel tired, sluggish, unfocused, and low on energy. You may even take a nap. You almost certainly do not feel full of energy.

Some might think that eating a large meal, thus supplying the body with an abundance of glucose, must be a good thing. Well, it's not that simple. The problem with overeating is simply an oversupply of glucose. Yes, you are providing sufficient glucose to all of the body's cells, but there is still a lot of glucose left circulating in the blood from that heavy meal, and it has nowhere to go. It makes sense that too little glucose in the body can be harmful (cells cannot function and you eventually fall into a coma!), but too much glucose in the body can also be harmful (diabetes is characterized by high blood glucose).

Our bodies are designed to resolve excessive amounts of glucose in the blood and return blood glucose to normal. However, finding cells able to accommodate the excess glucose and delivering it to them is a demanding process, and we tend to feel tired, sluggish, and generally lacking in energy while our body does this work. (And, just for the record, most of the excess glucose is stored as fat.)

How do you feel, on the other hand, when you have gone too long without eating? You probably feel tired, shaky, light-headed, irritable, moody, and, once again, low on energy. What is happening in your body to make your feel this way? The symptoms of eating too much and going too long without food are similar, but the causes are quite different.

In the case of going too long without eating, the reason for low energy is quite simple. Remember, food is fuel for the body. Specifically, the fuel is glucose, and in simple terms the food we consume is broken down to glucose, then transported in the blood to the body's cells, where it is metabolized to produce energy.

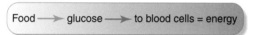

Food ⟶ glucose ⟶ to blood cells = energy

When we go too long without eating, then, we reduce the supply of glucose to the cells, and with less glucose available, less energy can be produced. In short: no glucose, no energy. But there's more. Our bodies are designed to adapt and survive, and, as a consequence, if we supply too little glucose, our body must and will do all it can to conserve energy. Thus our metabolism slows down, and all nonessential functions of the body are essentially switched off. As a result, we feel tired, sluggish, and irritable.

In contrast, eating light and often is a perfect strategy for managing the body's glucose supply; it ensures that we never have too much or too little glucose and, as a result, that we sustain a high energy level. So, how often should you eat?

We recommend that you eat approximately every 3 hours, give or take 1 hour, and that you never go longer than 4 hours without eating. In practical terms, we suggest three meals (breakfast, lunch, dinner) and two snacks daily. Never skip breakfast! Have at least a glass of juice or milk or a snack bar. Anything is better than nothing! You must consume something within 1 hour of waking. Remember, since you do not eat while sleeping, your glucose level is low when you awake in the morning.

If you eat three meals and two snacks a day, what would a typical schedule look like? Here is a sample:

Time	Meal
7:00 a.m.	Breakfast
10:30 a.m.	Snack
1:00 p.m.	Lunch
4:30 p.m.	Snack
7:00 p.m.	Dinner

You might wonder if snacks aren't unhealthy. Indeed, most of us have been taught for years to avoid snacks between meals, and you may have heard various reasons for this advice: "Snacks take away your appetite for meals," or "To lose weight, just eliminate snacks." In fact, these lines of thinking have now been exposed as faulty. Let's think about it in terms of glucose and energy. They key to sustaining a high level of energy is to maintain a healthy glucose supply, and, to this end, we have learned that you should never go longer than 4 hours without eating. How much time is there between your breakfast and lunch? Between your lunch and your dinner? If the interval is more than 4 hours, then you need to resupply your body with glucose, and that's where snacks come in. They provide a small but sufficient amount of glucose to help you maintain your energy.

The perfect snack is low-glycemic and provides approximately 100 to 150 calories (remember, this is not a meal, but just enough to get you there). Low-glycemic snacks are broken down more gradually into glucose than are high-glycemic foods, and they can provide energy for up to 2 hours (meals will always be low-glycemic if you follow our rules). In general, foods that contain protein, fiber, or fat in addition to carbohydrate tend to be low-glycemic. Examples include an energy bar with protein (but watch the calories and perhaps eat just half) or half of a whole-wheat bagel with peanut butter or cream cheese.

Frequently Asked Questions

Q: Healthy snacks are just not available at our workplace; in fact, we have nothing other than the typical snack machine filled with high-glycemic (and salty) snacks, soda, and coffee. Plus, someone always seems to bring in doughnuts, bagels, or cheesecake to share. What can I do?

A: We remember one attendee at our facility in Orlando who set a specific goal of getting a small fridge by Friday—and he did. He figured out that he'd have to shop for healthy snacks at the grocery store at least once a week and keep them in the small refrigerator in his office. Years later, it's still there, and it has solved his problem of lacking access to healthy snacks.

Other examples include yogurt, milk, a nutrition shake, mozzarella cheese, fruit (e.g., apple, orange, grapefruit, peach, pear), nuts, seeds, and hard-boiled eggs.

High-glycemic snacks, in contrast, are broken down rapidly and do not provide the sustained energy you want. You'll get a quick burst of energy followed by a rapid drop that leaves you feeling worse than you did before the snack. Avoid or limit these common high-glycemic snacks: plain bagels, sports drinks, breads low in fiber, cereals low in fiber, pretzels, and soda.

This is a good place to address a few typical mistakes people make. First, a large proportion of people begin their day without feeding their body any nutrients—that is, they skip breakfast. Somehow they expect to start the day working on leftover calories from the night before, and to mask the lack of fuel they may rely on coffee, diet soda, or other stimulants to get them moving. This approach results in a slow start and a late-morning energy slump that can be almost debilitating. If you feel like a typical breakfast is just not for you, then at least consume a healthy snack of 100 to 150 calories as your first meal of the day. It's best to make this snack a low-glycemic one; toaster pastries and doughnuts don't qualify.

Some people who skip breakfast increase the stress on their bodies by working out first thing in the morning. Thus they are trying to spend energy and calories that are just not available. Working out in the early morning is difficult enough for most people, and trying to do it without fuel is sure to discourage all but a hardy few. Remember, exercise requires glucose, and your glucose level is very low when you first get up. (You did not eat while you were asleep.) If sufficient glucose is not available, then your body must find fuel elsewhere to power the workout; unfortunately, this means breaking down lean muscle. So make sure you give your body at least some glucose—even a small glass of juice will do—then have your breakfast after the workout.

PhotoDisc

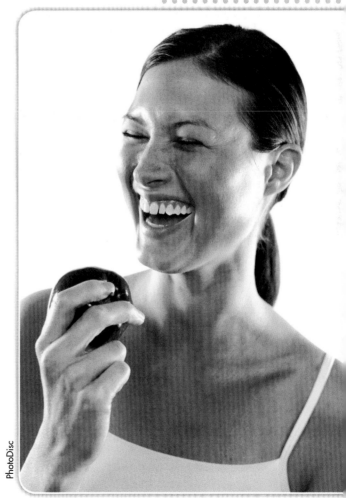

Healthy snacks will put a smile on your face.

A second pattern practiced by many people is to skip or go light on breakfast, then go light on lunch. By dinnertime, they are starved, and they proceed to make up for all the calories they should have consumed during the day, including too many want foods, then fall into a stupor in front of the television by early evening. This process, called "back-loading," is a self-defeating way to seek the fuel you need for energy during the day. Not only does it fail to meet your energy needs during the day, but it also collects a lot of useless calories that you don't need for sleep.

Eating similarly sized meals at breakfast, lunch, and dinner tends to keep your energy level higher and more consistent. Eating too much food during a meal fills no physical need but forces your body to figure out what to do with all those extra calories. (Would you be upset to learn that they will be stored as extra fat for a rainy day? We thought you might be!)

PORTION CONTROL

Now, let's discuss in a bit more detail what and how much you should eat during breakfast, lunch, and dinner. We recommend that you follow the same rule at each meal: Imagine dividing your meal into three components: grains (e.g., rice, pasta, cereal, bread), fruits and vegetables, and protein (e.g., lean meat, dairy products, nuts). Aim for 40 percent grain, 40 percent fruits and vegetables, and 20 percent protein (see figure 3.1). That's 40/40/20. This approach provides the balanced, healthy nutrition that is essential for optimal functioning of the body; it also provides you with sustained energy. Do not skimp on one of the food groups; if you do, you will compromise the *sustained energy* this approach promises.

One simple but effective way to measure how much you should eat is to use your hands, which, regardless of whether you are male or female, are generally proportional to your body size. Aim to eat no more than five handfuls of food

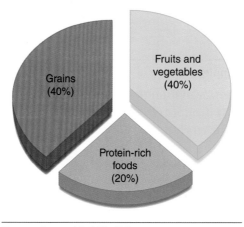

Figure 3.1 40/40/20 mix.

at each of your three meals: two handfuls of grain, two handfuls of fruits and vegetables, and one handful of protein. Cup one hand and imagine how much food you can hold in it (not a heaping cupful but a level one). That amount is one handful. For meat, use the palm of your hand as a gauge for the size and thickness that is appropriate (don't include the fingers and thumb). It's that simple! If you are a very active person, you should eat more often (including snacks) rather than increase the amount of food at mealtime.

For example, your breakfast could consist of two handfuls of cereal, one handful of fruit (such as chopped banana), a small glass of juice (i.e., another handful of fruit), and one handful of milk (for the cereal). Try applying the rule to a lunch or dinner meal for yourself. Table 3.1 shows a sample meal plan for two days.

Now, remember those want foods (e.g., desserts, fries, alcohol) and the four-to-one ratio of need versus want foods? Well, to improve your ratio, all you have to do is replace one handful of grain with one handful of want food. For example, if you want to include a glass of wine with dinner, reduce your grains by eliminating bread or rolls with that meal. As long as you adhere to this ratio, you will still get one handful of grain, and the want food will provide energy

TABLE 3.1　Sample Two-Day Meal Plan

	Day 1	Day 2
Breakfast	Half a toasted whole-wheat bagel with peanut butter (no sugar added) Small glass of fortified orange juice Half a banana Water	Muesli with milk Walnuts Berries Yogurt Water
Snack 1	Nutrition bar with protein and fiber Water	12 cashews Water
Lunch	Half a chicken salad sandwich with fresh spinach and tomatoes Vegetable-based soup Water	Whole-wheat pita Greek salad Hummus Water
Snack 2	Half an apple Milk 　OR 15 peanuts or almonds Water	Trail mix Water
Dinner	Salmon Green salad Rice Grilled vegetables 1 glass of wine Water	Grilled chicken Garlic spinach Mashed potatoes Dessert Water

too. This approach will help you meet your goal of sustaining high energy and enjoying foods you want. However, we recommend no more than two alcohol substitutions per day.

A note about supplements: Many folks spend a lot of time trying to figure out whether to add nutritional supplements to their diets. We believe that a healthy, balanced diet is by far the most important factor in providing energy and that if you follow our guidelines for proportions of different food groups you'll more than satisfy your nutritional needs. At most, we would suggest that you consider a daily multivitamin if you are not able to consistently adhere to these guidelines. Beyond that, we urge you to consult your personal physician or a certified nutritionist for special needs or circumstances.

If you are interested in a thorough treatment of nutrition, we strongly recommend the following books:

- *Nancy Clark's Sports Nutrition Guidebook, Fourth Edition* (2008, Human Kinetics, Champaign, IL)
- *The Anti-Diet Book,* by Jack Groppel (1997, Human Performance Institute, Orlando, FL)

LOSING WEIGHT

Most of us gain some weight each year as life goes on. While the increase often accumulates slowly, we may realize in middle age that more than a few pounds have sneaked up on us. If this is your situation, you are not alone: About two-thirds of Americans are overweight, and half of these are obese. This is one of the highest rates in the world, and the numbers are likely to get worse since weight gain during childhood has nearly tripled in the United States over the last 20 years.

Often, our first response to being overweight is to go on a diet, and you might wonder whether the nutrition tips we recommend in this chapter just amount to another diet. Our emphatic answer is no. Instead, what we are proposing is a lifestyle change in nutrition habits that will maximize your personal energy and give your body the fuel you need in order to function at an optimal level. If you follow the guidelines outlined in this chapter, we're confident that you'll establish daily rituals that allow you to enjoy food, fuel your body, and have energy to burn.

In addition, if you adopt our eating strategies, then the timing, nutrient content, and portion sizes of your eating will maximize your opportunity to lose body fat. If you combine these eating strategies with an equally sound plan for regular physical activity, the chances for you to lose weight are excellent. Remember that what we're measuring is not just weight loss but your percentage of body fat as compared with that of muscle and of bone.

HYDRATION AND BEVERAGES

Finally, let's discuss beverages. The most important beverage is water—an essential nutrient that helps maintain optimal functioning of the body. Water is essential for transporting nutrients to cells and removing metabolic by-products from cells. The evaporation of water also helps cool the body and maintain a consistent body temperature even during exercise.

Suggestions abound about how much water we should drink daily, but in reality people's water needs vary, and we recommend that you have water available and sip it regularly throughout the day. Most people consume less than half of the optimal amount of water each day, so try doubling your current water intake to start.

Some folks count intake of other beverages toward their daily water consumption goals, but we think this approach is a bit risky. Most drinks contain other ingredients, such as caffeine or sugar, and many are high-glycemic. We suggest that you stick to water when monitoring daily fluid intake.

If you exercise and perspire, especially in hot weather, you need to increase your fluid intake before, during, and after activity in order to replace lost fluids. Your body cools itself by dissipating excess heat through sweating, and sports drinks can be helpful during and after activity since they replace carbohydrate lost through activity while also maintaining optimal levels of sodium and potassium in your body. Remember, however, that sports drinks are typically high in sugar and calories and that you probably do not need all the sugar they provide. Diluting sports drinks at a ratio of one to one (one part sports drink, one part water) will help you rehydrate and replace carbohydrate, sodium, and potassium without consuming an excessive number of calories.

High-calorie beverages such as soda are considered want foods and are best managed if you consume them with

PhotoDisc

It's important to maintain good hydration all day long.

meals and substitute them for a handful of grain. Diet soda without calories appears to be a smart substitute for regular sodas, but the long-term effects of sugar substitutes on the body are still not understood. If you drink diet soft drinks, do so with meals and limit them to one or two per day.

Finally, we come to alcohol, which is also a want food and should also be substituted for a grain at a meal if you choose to consume it. We recommend that you consume no more than two servings of alcohol each day. If you exceed this amount, the calories consumed will throw the balance of your hard work off kilter, and before long the extra weight will begin to show up. A serving is one 12-ounce beer, one 1.5-ounce shot of hard alcohol (such as whisky or vodka), or one 5-ounce glass of wine.

While you can technically substitute a regular soda or an alcoholic beverage for a grain and still manage your energy, we urge you to remember that grains in your meal provide important nutrients. Try to limit your consumption of regular sodas and alcohol.

Jim works in computer software sales; he travels during most weeks and arrives home on Friday nights. As he travels, most evenings require him to entertain clients for dinner. A typical schedule includes meeting for drinks before dinner, ordering wine during dinner, and finishing the evening with an after-dinner drink. Although Jim knows he should cut down on his alcohol consumption, he feels that social custom almost demands that he use alcohol to relax with a prospective client, forge good feelings, and seem like an okay guy. If Jim continues this pattern, what are the likely consequences of his alcohol consumption? What solution should he consider to reduce his alcohol intake?

Possible solution: This all-too-common situation puts Jim in the difficult position of consuming significantly more than the daily recommended amount of alcohol. Possible outcomes include ingesting empty calories (calories with no nutritional content), exceeding the recommended five handfuls of food at one meal, and potentially developing a dependence on alcohol that could become a chronic issue. We'd suggest first that Jim start out by socializing before dinner with a nonalcoholic drink, such as water, mineral water, or, if desired, sparkling water flavored with lemon or lime. If he chooses an alcoholic beverage, he should do so *during* dinner, when he is also ingesting food, thus lessening the effect of alcohol. Remember that a glass of wine or beer can be substituted for one serving of grain if you are adhering to the guideline of eating five handfuls for portion control. Finally, we'd eliminate the after-dinner drink; again, a nonalcoholic beverage will work just fine.

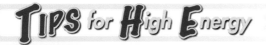

TIPS for High Energy

- Eat three meals and two snacks daily.
- Eat light and often.
- Never skip breakfast; begin the day with at least a snack.
- Make sure you eat a balanced diet at each meal by using the following proportions: 40 percent grain, 40 percent fruits and vegetables, and 20 percent protein.
- Limit your total portions at each meal to five handfuls or less.
- Never go longer than 4 hours without food.
- Drink water regularly and increase fluid consumption before, during, and after physical activity.
- Limit alcohol to one or two servings per day.

CHAPTER 4

MOTIVATING YOURSELF FOR PHYSICAL ACTIVITY

We won't kid you. It can be challenging to change from a sedentary lifestyle to one that includes daily physical activity. It might help you to think about the challenge in this way:

A challenge is simply a stimulating task or problem that presents various obstacles. A challenge also provides an opportunity for positive change and growth.

Many challenges involve a lack of cognitive understanding as well as insufficient emotional commitment to change our behavior. We often describe this state as simply a lack of motivation, and perhaps it is. But sometimes even when we do have motivation, it is not powerful enough to support lasting change. So how can we generate more powerful motivation?

This chapter helps you understand the importance and power of motivation if you are to bring about lasting behavioral change. It also helps you understand how internal motivation flowing from your deepest values is more powerful than depending on external motivators. We suggest specific strategies to increase your motivation to engage in physical activity; we want you to feel pulled—not pushed—toward a physically active lifestyle. We also discuss stress and recovery. Most of us know that too much stress is unhealthy, but we want you to regard stress as a potentially positive force in moving you toward high performance, as long as you also make time for recovery from stress. Physical activity can be a powerful ally in the recovery phase; it helps you reenergize your mind, body, and spirit to face the next challenge.

GETTING MOTIVATED FOR CHANGE

Simply defined, "motivation is the direction of effort and the intensity of effort" (Weinberg and Gould 2007). To become motivated to be physically active, you must invest *effort* and *energy* into the process.

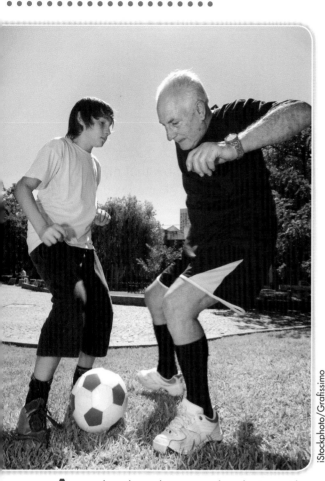

A grandpa shows his energy by playing with his grandson.

iStockphoto/Grafissimo

Psychologists have drawn a distinction between extrinsic and intrinsic motivation, and the difference resides in the source. Extrinsic motivation comes from outside of ourselves—for example, from a spouse, parents, a child, a boss, friends, or others who offer positive or negative reinforcement of our actions. Extrinsic rewards include money, status, recognition by others, awards, and other tangible benefits such as a night out to celebrate an accomplishment. Although such rewards can be helpful in pushing us toward change, they are nowhere near as powerful as intrinsic motivation that comes from deep within our own mind and personality.

Intrinsic, or internal, motivation involves a feeling within a person that is directed toward becoming a competent, self-determining, and successful self. People who are internally motivated dream, set their own goals, expend great effort toward achievement, and, at the end of the day, are rewarded by the knowledge that they worked hard, embraced the challenge, and did their best.

As compared with intrinsic rewards, extrinsic rewards bestowed by others may provide an incentive in the short term, but the effect eventually subsides. Ultimately, extrinsic rewards are superficial and transient, and often they do not connect to your deepest values and beliefs. Thus, starting a physical activity program and rewarding yourself with a shopping spree for new clothes may not be as effective as starting the program in order to be more active and energetic with your grandchildren. With more energy, you can look forward to many years of nurturing a close connection with those grandkids.

Keep this difference in mind when planning your program for physical activity. We don't totally discount the value of extrinsic motivators, and we recognize that they may be helpful in the short term, but without deeper intrinsic motivators your ability to sustain long-term change will be compromised. In the final analysis, *your* feelings count more than those of others when you evaluate your progress and your success or failure to perform.

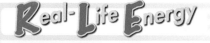

Real-Life Energy

It's been 2 years since I completed the Corporate Athlete Course. I am 39 years old and have often had peaks and valleys in both my exercise and my eating habits. I would get serious about diet and exercise, then over a period of time lose motivation (purpose) and fall back into old habits. Now, after almost 2 years, I have exercised at least 5 days a week and had maybe 2 days of not eating within a 4-hour period. I feel amazing! I know that my productivity, stress level, and energy throughout the day have all improved significantly. I have lost 40 pounds (18 kilograms) and know when I haven't had enough water because my body is quick to tell me. What's even better is that I wake up ready for my workout and then feel amazing all day, giving my best to both my family and employer. I recently did my health risk assessment and have phenomenal numbers!

Saying I have had success doesn't mean there haven't been challenges, too. When I do "slide," I quickly get myself back in gear. It's not so hard to do, because I know now how good I feel when I'm at my highest energy peak.

—Valerie Dinges, manager, GlaxoSmithKline

Get yourself ready for positive change by programming your mind with private thoughts that are positive, affirming, and geared toward taking action now. This type of self-talk can become your mantra. In the following examples, notice the difference between the negative self-talk in the left column and the more positive phrases on the right. The negative phrases will lead only to feelings of anger, frustration, or helplessness and set you up for failure, whereas the positive ones are energizing and hopeful.

Negative self-talk	Positive self-talk
I've got to do it.	I want to.
I should do it.	I can do this.
Others expect me to.	It would be fun to do.
It's good for me.	It would feel good.
I know I should, but . . .	I'm ready to do it.

You can see the power of emphasizing intrinsic motivation based on your most deeply held beliefs and values to pull you toward your goals. During the process of changing your behavior, it is useful to monitor the voice in your head that initiates self-talk and comments on your ability to succeed and on the change process itself. Think of yourself as a positive, affirming self-coach who looks for good things to say along the way. An oft-repeated positive thought tends to become a self-fulfilling prophecy that helps you move in your desired direction.

To make a significant change in your behavior, think of this formula:

cognitive change → emotional investment → physical action

If you want to add more physical activity to your life, you need to read about the benefits, options, and barriers and learn as much as you can about the subject, just as you are doing now. That's the cognitive or mental side of getting started. Think of it as planning a great adventure. Next, you need to invest emotional energy in the decision to make some changes in your lifestyle. Your emotions fuel the change process. Embrace energy-producing emotions such as excitement, passion, and hope. Finally, you've got to take the physical steps, such as investigating exercise facilities, securing equipment and clothing, and developing a schedule to get you started. We address specifics of these steps in greater detail throughout the book. Right now, it is important just to understand the process. If you skip any of these three steps—the mental, the emotional, the physical—you will be wasting well-intentioned effort. Start with your mind, add strong feelings, and take action. That's the formula right there.

CHANGE AS A 4-STAGE PROCESS

In order to move from an inactive lifestyle to an active one, it may be helpful to think in terms of four distinct stages:

- Stage 1: You are inactive but thinking about physical activity.
- Stage 2: You are doing some physical activity but probably not with the frequency, intensity, or duration that would be best for your health.
- Stage 3: You are physically active at a good level.
- Stage 4: You have integrated the habit of being physically active into your lifestyle.

Let's assume that you are now at stage 1. What should you do to move toward stage 2?

Stage 1 Actions: Think, Visualize, and Remove Barriers

First, read anything you can get your hands on that extols the virtues of physical activity. Pay attention to the health benefits, the effect on personal energy, the fun, the social contacts, the positive feelings that activity can generate. Picture yourself, sweating, after an activity session, enjoying a feeling of energy, well-being, and satisfaction.

Frank is a financial analyst who works for a large company. As the economy has stumbled through some down years, business has not been good, and there's been talk of a possible merger or acquisition of his company.

At midlife, Frank and his wife Carol have three children under the age of 15, and Carol works part-time. Just keeping up with their busy life and that of three kids provides challenge enough. Yet Frank works long hours and feels increasing pressure to produce new business. He can't afford to change careers at this stage, and the fear of starting over again with a new company is daunting. Family expenses are under control, but the mortgage, cars, vacations, and looming college expenses leave little room for error.

On a typical workday, Frank leaves home at 7 a.m. and returns about 7 p.m. Usually he's exhausted and wants time to unwind with a drink; he then checks his e-mail and voice messages and watches the evening news. After dinner, he checks to see that homework assignments have been done and often falls asleep in front of the television. It seems that there's just no time in his schedule for physical activity except on weekends. Even then, he often feels lethargic and just wants some rest to recharge for the next cycle of work.

Is there hope for Frank to break out of this pattern of physical inactivity? To create more personal energy?

Frank's situation is exactly the type that can be changed productively by following a plan to create new priorities, a personal commitment to change, and daily rituals to achieve a more physically active life. His problem is not lack of time; it is lack of a commitment to raising his personal energy and thus enabling himself to become fully engaged throughout long days at work and afterward with his family at home. It can be done, and we address the specifics in the coming chapters.

Second, contemplate the typical hindrances to activity and be creative in coming up with solutions. Here are the most commonly reported obstacles to physical activity:

- *Time.* "I just don't have time. Life is too busy, other obligations take priority, and there are not enough hours in the day."
- *Lack of partners.* "I'd like to try a sport or activity, but I can't find a partner or buddy to join me. You can't play tennis or basketball alone, and I like social sports."
- *Lack of skill.* "I wish I were better at sports, but basically I played team sports. Now I wish I had the skills to do individual lifetime sports that I could do at any age."
- *Lack of energy.* "It sounds funny, but after a full day of work, I'm just too tired to even think about activity. I need to just relax and rest up for the next day."

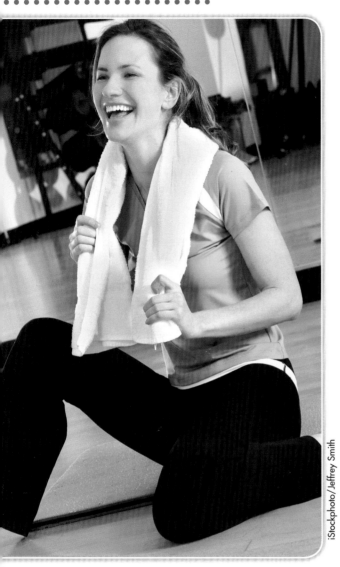

iStockphoto/Jeffrey Smith

Picture yourself as happy, with a sense of accomplishment after physical activity.

- *Money.* "The physical activities I'd like to try are just too expensive. Our priorities are for our children's education, family vacations, and retirement. Going skiing, joining a gym, or playing golf is out of our reach financially."

- *Injury.* "I'd like to be more active, but my back has been a problem for years. And the stress on my back has now affected my knees and hips. I'm not very flexible and probably would injure myself if I tried a new activity."

- *Work.* "Our business is a bottom-line one, and my boss expects me to work long hours pretty much every week. If I take time to be active, I'm sure he'd think I am slacking off."

- *Family.* "I feel like any spare time I have should be devoted to my spouse and kids. After all, they are the most important thing in the world to me, and I rarely get to spend time with them. Exercising seems so selfish, like I'm more important than they are."

- *Health issues.* "I've had some health scares lately, and I've got to just take care of myself and not stress my body too much. Even though my doctor has cleared me for activity, I'm afraid to risk it."

There may be more excuses, but this list includes the ones we hear most often. As you read them over, can you see possible solutions to any of them? If not, discuss them with someone who is physically active to see how he or she has handled the same apparent barriers. If you believe you have other barriers, make a list of them and brainstorm or talk with others about potential solutions.

We revisit these issues in chapter 11 and offer our own suggestions for resolving them. And if you need help in overcoming these barriers just to get started, we give you permission to peek into chapter 11 now!

Stage 2 Actions: Increase the Frequency, Duration, and Intensity of Activity

In stage 2, you are doing some physical activity but not at the needed frequency, intensity, or duration. Let's look at relevant factors and set some goals.

The *frequency* of physical activity needs to be at least three times a week, and the *duration* should be 60 minutes per session (Centers for Disease Control and Prevention 2008). Better yet, set your ultimate goal at five times a week (thus allowing two rest days).

Be sure that the time you allocate to physical activity includes time for warm-up and dynamic stretching at the beginning, as well as cool-down and static stretching at the end. Failure to treat your body kindly before and after activity can easily lead to injury or frustrating soreness. At a minimum, we suggest 10 minutes of warm-up and dynamic stretching, 45 minutes of workout activity, and 5 minutes of cool-down and static stretching.

If a lack of time is holding you back from following this schedule, look for ways to reduce other commitments. Consider early morning activity, lunch breaks, or early evenings—and of course weekends. Some people who are unable to be physically active for 60 minutes at a time have managed to integrate two 30-minute periods or even four 15-minute segments during the workday. Continuous physical activity for 60 minutes is optimal, but shorter segments can be effective.

The *intensity* of physical activity is measured best by assessing your heart rate. You can do so most accurately by purchasing a heart rate monitor (for less than $50 in the United States) and wearing it during activity. If this method is inappropriate for your type of activity or sport, you can take your pulse for 15 seconds and multiply that number by 4 to get a fairly accurate idea of your heart rate. Some fitness machines in gyms measure your heart rate for you.

Your objective for your heart rate is to elevate it into a "training zone," which is calculated in the following manner: Subtract your age from 220 to calculate your maximum heart rate. For example, let's say that you are 40 years old: 220 − 40 (your age) = 180. Now, multiply the result (180) by 80 percent (0.8). The answer, 144, would be a good training zone for your heart. As you progress, you might want to train at 90 percent. If you are just beginning to intensify your physical activity, aim for 60 or 70 percent of your maximum for several weeks in order to acclimate your body to the stress of exertion. For example, for the 40-year-old in the preceding example, the calculated maximum heart rate is 180; if you multiply that figure by 60 percent (0.6), you arrive at an answer of 108. Raising one's heart rate to 108 is a moderate training level, and it is appropriate for a 40-year-old who is unaccustomed to physical activity.

Our experience has shown that committing yourself to achieving greater frequency, duration, and intensity is critical to improving your fitness and energy. *But you don't have to change all of these factors at once.* Instead, we suggest that you increase at least one of the factors each week, keep a record of your progress, and advance gradually until you are meeting the standards we have laid out here.

One last thought on strengthening your performance at stage 2: Reward and celebrate your success with each improvement you make. Reconnect with the intrinsic goals you have set, such as becoming more energetic and active with your kids or grandkids. Another part of celebrating your success is to give yourself a verbal pat on the back in the form of positive self-talk. Helpful phrases ("I'm on my way," "This feels good," "I'm getting faster and stronger," "Way to go!") should flow easily at this point. You might also try a little extrinsic motivation by telling others about your progress, indulging yourself with a tangible reward such as new sports or activity equipment, or enjoying an unrelated reward such as seeing a show or movie. Each time you reinforce your positive progress, you will strengthen your resolve and motivate yourself for more success.

Stage 3 Actions: Sustain and Move to Stage 4

If you've succeeded at moving into stage 3—in which your level of physical activity meets your goals for frequency, duration, and intensity—what's next? For one thing, you'd like to sustain that level of activity even when obstacles appear.

Our experience shows that people often have to overcome obstacles caused by illness, injury, or a family- or work-related crisis. Each of these life events can undercut the progress you have made. In some cases, you'll have to adjust your activity routine to accommodate the outside stress by changing the activity, frequency, or intensity. But even if you need to make changes, we urge you to at least stay active on a maintenance program of physical activity. It's clear that in times of stress, physical activity is one of the best ways to relieve tension and restore your body to a healthier state.

If you do encounter obstacles, you are somewhat at risk for losing sight of your original motivation for becoming physically active. This is the time to return to your strongest motivators for activity and renew them intellectually and emotionally. Develop self-talk habits that reflect your new challenges and affirm your positive approach to confronting them: "I've done it before and I can do it again." "One step at a time—I'm getting better every day." "I'm on the right path."

Stage 4 Actions: Keep on Moving

At this level, physical activity has been so integrated into your life that it simply can't be removed except by a severe illness or injury. By this time, you have gained experience in identifying everyday obstacles that arise, finding solutions, and strengthening your resolve. The fact that you've been buffeted by obstacles and have overcome them boosts your confidence in yourself to do so again.

Physical activity at stage 4 has become an automatic part of your life, just like eating and sleeping. It takes little thought, because you've absolutely committed to a life of activity, and daily physical movement is a ritual that you integrate into each day. Our only caution is that you might plan ahead by trying new physical activities that could become useful in the future. Having a variety of skills and interests and being familiar with several forms of physical activity gives you a better chance of sustaining your level in spite of obstacles that may pop up. We also encourage you to reach out to an increasingly wider circle of friends and acquaintances to expand your physical activity circle. Each new person brings a fresh approach to activity, and he or she may become a candidate for social friendship as well.

At this fourth stage, your motivation for physical activity is no longer an issue, but it makes sense not to take a good thing for granted. We suggest that you indulge in a short gratitude exercise, during which you express your thankfulness for the opportunity to be physically active. Take a few minutes to write down why you find physical activity so satisfying, enriching, and energizing and express your gratitude for the fact that you are able to enjoy it. Many people don't know the joy and exhilaration that physical activity can bring even in the later decades of life.

EMBRACING STRESS AND RECOVERY CYCLES

One of the great dilemmas we face today is handling the stress that seems to build up in our lives. It may derive from, among other sources, work, overall schedule, family issues, finances, relationships, shortage of time, or health problems. When you feel stressed, a voice in your head may tell you to simply ignore it and hope it will go away. Meanwhile, lectures, books, and seminars purport to tell us how to deal with stress mainly by avoiding it or adopting behaviors that mask its effects.

We'd like to suggest, instead, that you *embrace* stress. Think of it as something powerful that can help you accomplish goals that previously seemed unreachable. Feelings of stress can help energize you to expend your maximum effort and accomplish much. Great challenges in life usually involve great stress, doubt, and uncertainty that end in success if you smartly *invest energy toward the perceived obstacles*.

Think of training a muscle for strength and endurance. It happens not by accident but only through expenditure of energy through exercise, overload, and multiple repetitions. You simply can't gain strength unless you stress the muscle.

Likewise, in other areas of your life (e.g., work), stress can be a powerful force to help you achieve goals you may have thought impossible. Most people are at least somewhat fearful of making public speeches or presentations, for example, yet the opportunity to do so may force you to prepare thoroughly, clarify your thoughts, and present a persuasive argument in order to convince others to share your point of view. Once the ordeal is over, the exultation that flows from your success can produce a great feeling of satisfaction and boost your self-confidence.

We've got to admit, however, that too much stress can be debilitating. Our minds, emotions, and physical bodies need periods of rest and recovery from stress. In fact, for many of us, recovery time is the key factor that we ignore in the race to get ahead in life. But recovery cycles are the time when *growth* occurs (see figure 4.1). Muscles grow during rest periods, and the same is true in our mental and emotional dimensions. Rest cycles allow us to replenish our energy in order to handle the next stressor that is certain to appear. They are critical to the high performance that all competitive athletes seek, and the most successful competitors have learned to schedule rest and relaxation cycles after periods of intense training.

Physical activity itself can become a key recovery strategy for you. When you are bothered by the weight of work responsibilities, family obligations, or financial worries, physical exercise can help you clear your mind and refocus your thoughts, especially if you choose a physical activity that is fun for you. The break from work will be a pleasant and invigorating respite from your daily routine, and, by stimulating production of serotonin in your brain, physical activity will enhance your mood and help you feel better about yourself.

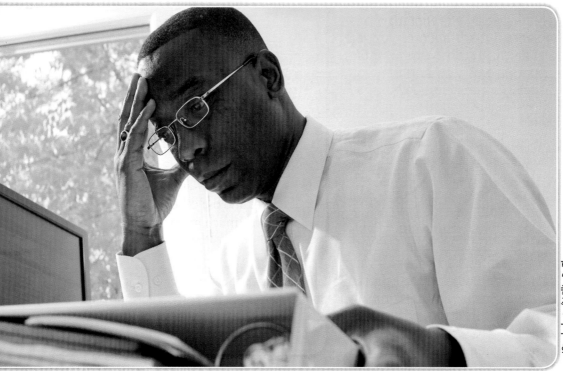

iStockphoto/Willie B. Thomas

Stress can be positive or negative, depending on how you deal with it.

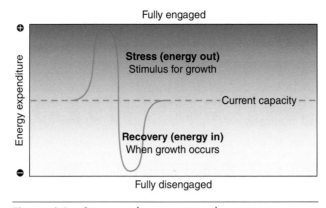

Fully engaged

Stress (energy out)
Stimulus for growth

Current capacity

Recovery (energy in)
When growth occurs

Fully disengaged

Figure 4.1 Stress and recovery cycles.

The key to dealing with stress, then, is to embrace it and use it to achieve your highest goals while also building in time for recovery by respecting the natural cycle of stress and recovery. During your recovery time, use physical activity to clear your mind, relax your body, and change your mood. Taking care of your physical dimension will help you feel healthier, more energetic, and ready to deal with the next stressful incident that is bound to appear in your life.

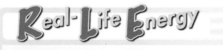

Members of the Harbor Beach Marriott executive team attended the Corporate Athlete Course at the Human Performance Institute in 2008 and enjoyed a team-building experience they will never forget. In the hospitality business, it is important to make sure that things run smoothly 24 hours a day, 7 days a week. "It inevitably adds a bit of pressure for all team members to make themselves available 24-7," says area general manager Jim Mauer.

Before attending the course, team members felt guilty about taking time off to exercise, go on vacation, or just take a break. "This training opened our eyes to the importance of taking care of ourselves and our other employees," says Mauer. He explains that his team has become much more supportive of one another. In fact, "we've noticed a change in people's attitudes, commitment, and engagement levels." In one year, the team's customer rating has improved from a score of 77 to 86.5, and the associate rating of the executive team has increased by 8 points (from 73 to 81)—a great improvement in the hospitality industry. The next step for this team is to train its 77 managers and 800 staff members to integrate their new knowledge into their work in meetings, restaurants, and the fitness center and spa—for the benefit of both consumers and staff.

Think of your life as a series of peaks and valleys that symbolize stress and recovery cycles. Stress requires that you expend energy, and recovery requires that you renew your energy and capacity for exertion. You must build both into your daily routine in order to maximize your performance, health, and happiness. The lesson here is that even as you move into a more physically active lifestyle, you must remember to allow equal time for recovery—physically, emotionally, and mentally.

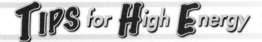

- Changing your lifestyle is a challenge for you to embrace.
- Motivation from within yourself is the most powerful tool you possess.
- Identify potential obstacles to physical activity and propose solutions.
- Moving from stage 1 to stage 4 in your commitment to physical activity requires knowledge, understanding, commitment, and clear goals against which to measure progress.
- Stress can be good for you, but only if you also make time for rest and recovery.

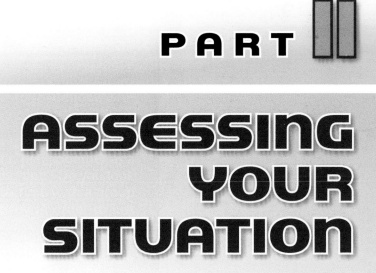

PART II

ASSESSING YOUR SITUATION

CHAPTER 5

DETERMINING YOUR HEALTH AND FITNESS LEVELS

The first key step toward enhancing your personal energy level is to honestly assess your current levels of health and fitness. If you have been kidding yourself about your fitness, this is the time to take a realistic look. Doing so will set your starting point and help you develop a personal prescription tailored to your fitness level, age, sex, and specific strengths and weaknesses.

Identifying your current health and fitness levels helps you establish a baseline against which to mark your progress as you increase your physical activity. As you start to see improvement, your motivation will increase, you'll gain confidence that you are on the right track, and you can reward yourself for success. If, on the other hand, retesting at prescribed intervals shows that you are not progressing as you had hoped, you will know that it is time to make adjustments in your activity.

Before you embark on any physical activity program, it is essential to get medical clearance and make sure that you are safely able to start. In this chapter, we discuss how to get the clearance you need and how to assess your current health and fitness level through simple tests. This process prepares you for your physical activity program and allows you to measure your progress.

INITIAL HEALTH ASSESSMENT

The first order of business is to be sure that your medical doctor understands your commitment to increasing your level of physical activity and gives you the green light to proceed. In fact, it's a good idea to have a complete medical examination by a physician before you begin. If you face medical limitations, such as joint weakness, high blood pressure, medication issues, or other concerns, this is the time for your doctor to caution you, suggest warning signs, and perhaps modify your activity plan.

We also suggest that before beginning any physical activity program, you complete the checklist shown in figure 5.1 and consult your doctor for his or her recommendations based on your answers.

Physical Activity Readiness
Questionnaire - PAR-Q
(revised 2002)

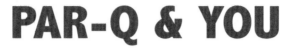

PAR-Q & YOU

(A Questionnaire for People Aged 15 to 69)

Regular physical activity is fun and healthy, and increasingly more people are starting to become more active every day. Being more active is very safe for most people. However, some people should check with their doctor before they start becoming much more physically active.

If you are planning to become much more physically active than you are now, start by answering the seven questions in the box below. If you are between the ages of 15 and 69, the PAR-Q will tell you if you should check with your doctor before you start. If you are over 69 years of age, and you are not used to being very active, check with your doctor.

Common sense is your best guide when you answer these questions. Please read the questions carefully and answer each one honestly: check YES or NO.

YES	NO		
☐	☐	**1.**	**Has your doctor ever said that you have a heart condition <u>and</u> that you should only do physical activity recommended by a doctor?**
☐	☐	**2.**	**Do you feel pain in your chest when you do physical activity?**
☐	☐	**3.**	**In the past month, have you had chest pain when you were not doing physical activity?**
☐	☐	**4.**	**Do you lose your balance because of dizziness or do you ever lose consciousness?**
☐	☐	**5.**	**Do you have a bone or joint problem (for example, back, knee or hip) that could be made worse by a change in your physical activity?**
☐	☐	**6.**	**Is your doctor currently prescribing drugs (for example, water pills) for your blood pressure or heart condition?**
☐	☐	**7.**	**Do you know of <u>any other reason</u> why you should not do physical activity?**

If

you

answered

YES to one or more questions

Talk with your doctor by phone or in person BEFORE you start becoming much more physically active or BEFORE you have a fitness appraisal. Tell your doctor about the PAR-Q and which questions you answered YES.

- You may be able to do any activity you want — as long as you start slowly and build up gradually. Or, you may need to restrict your activities to those which are safe for you. Talk with your doctor about the kinds of activities you wish to participate in and follow his/her advice.
- Find out which community programs are safe and helpful for you.

NO to all questions

If you answered NO honestly to <u>all</u> PAR-Q questions, you can be reasonably sure that you can:
- start becoming much more physically active – begin slowly and build up gradually. This is the safest and easiest way to go.
- take part in a fitness appraisal – this is an excellent way to determine your basic fitness so that you can plan the best way for you to live actively. It is also highly recommended that you have your blood pressure evaluated. If your reading is over 144/94, talk with your doctor before you start becoming much more physically active.

DELAY BECOMING MUCH MORE ACTIVE:
- if you are not feeling well because of a temporary illness such as a cold or a fever – wait until you feel better; or
- if you are or may be pregnant – talk to your doctor before you start becoming more active.

PLEASE NOTE: If your health changes so that you then answer YES to any of the above questions, tell your fitness or health professional. Ask whether you should change your physical activity plan.

<u>Informed Use of the PAR-Q</u>: The Canadian Society for Exercise Physiology, Health Canada, and their agents assume no liability for persons who undertake physical activity, and if in doubt after completing this questionnaire, consult your doctor prior to physical activity.

No changes permitted. You are encouraged to photocopy the PAR-Q but only if you use the entire form.

Figure 5.1   PAR-Q.

Source: *Physical Activity Readiness Questionnaire (PAR-Q)* © 2002. Used with permission from the Canadian Society for Exercise Physiology www.csep.ca.

SELF-TESTS FOR FITNESS

Many fitness test options are available, and our suggestions for you are designed to be simple, easy to carry out, inexpensive, and scientifically sound. If you choose to work with a physical trainer or other fitness coach, he or she may recommend other tests that will give you similar information. It is crucial, however, that once you choose a set of fitness tests, you continue to use them to track your progress. If you use the same tests, in a fashion identical to that of your initial testing, then you can use retesting to accurately assess your progress over time.

The four key factors in assessing physical fitness are as follows:

- Cardiorespiratory fitness (aerobic capacity)
- Muscular strength and endurance
- Flexibility
- Body composition

These four factors are the basic indicators of fitness for everyone. Each factor can be explored in depth and detail, but for your purposes now a general evaluation of each will provide an excellent starting point. Table 5.1 shows what assessment test is recommended for each component, as well as what equipment is needed for each test.

TABLE 5.1   Components, Assessment Tests, and Equipment

Fitness component	Assessment test	Equipment needed
Cardiorespiratory fitness (aerobic capacity)	Cooper test for 12 minutes	• Flat walking surface or running track (distance should be marked at intervals so that you can measure the distance run during the allotted time) • Stopwatch or watch with second hand
Muscular strength and endurance	Push-up maximum (without rest) followed by maximum number of sit-ups in 1 minute*	None
Flexibility	Sit-and-reach test	Yardstick and adhesive tape
Body composition	Body composition (percent body fat)	Access to equipment for measuring body composition

* Take a short rest period after the push-up test to allow yourself to feel comfortable before starting the sit-up test.

Options for measuring body composition include use of a Bod Pod, which measures air displacement; hydrostatic weighing, which measures water displacement; bioelectrical impedance analysis; and skinfold measurement with calipers. Of these, we prefer the Bod Pod for its accuracy, reliability, and relative comfort for the participant (see www.bodpod.com to locate the nearest Bod Pod testing location). As an alternative, bioelectrical impedance analysis (BIA) is quick, convenient, and inexpensive, and you can purchase your own BIA body fat analyzer for home use (see www.omron.com). BIA is not as accurate or reliable as measurement using a Bod Pod, but it can provide useful feedback on your progress. Most fitness centers offer this service, and your doctor may be able to recommend a convenient testing site. Once you choose a method, stick to it in order to minimize errors in assessment. We recommend that you measure regularly (perhaps once a week) under consistent conditions and look at the trend for your percent body fat.

These assessment methods assume that the body is made up of fat and nonfat components. The percent body fat measured is compared with norms established based on age and gender. Generally, a body fat percentage between 16 and 24 is considered average (at the 50th percentile) for men's health, and a percentage between 21 and 30 is considered average (at the 50th percentile) for women, depending on age. Of course, the most important comparison is to measure change in your percent body fat once you begin an activity program.

CARDIORESPIRATORY TEST

The cardiorespiratory test, also called the Cooper test (Cooper 1968), assesses the ability of your heart, lungs, and blood vessels to transport oxygen throughout your body. The more oxygen you can transport, the greater your cardiorespiratory fitness. For this test, we suggest that you wear comfortable clothing and athletic shoes that have been broken in. Avoid smoking, eating, or ingesting caffeine for at least 2 hours before you take the test.

➤ **Objective**   Run or walk as far as possible in 12 minutes.

➤ **Directions**

1. Warm up your body for 3 to 5 minutes by walking and doing jumping jacks and large stretching movements (e.g., trunk twists, reaching with your arms) to raise your body temperature, elevate your heart rate, and ready your muscles for activity. If possible, you should have practiced pacing prior to the test. People often attempt to run too fast early in the run and become fatigued prematurely.

2. If you are using a 440-yard track, place traffic cones or a similar marker every 88 yards on the inside edge of the first lane. The first marker should be placed at the starting line. If you are using a 400-meter track, markers are placed every 80 meters (87.5 yards) on the inside edge of the first lane. In either case, there should be a total of five markers placed on the track. If you are not using a track, you will have to measure the distances and place markers at the five positions described above. Make a note of your exact starting time.

3. Begin running at a pace that you believe you will be able to sustain for 12 minutes. If you need to slow down and walk, you may do so, though of course you will then cover less distance.

4. Stop running or walking when 12 minutes have passed. Record the number of markers you have passed during the 12 minutes. There are five cones per lap completed. If you finish at a point between markers, give yourself credit only for the last cone that you passed. If you are using a 440-yard track, multiply the number of cones you passed by 0.05 to obtain your distance in miles. If you are using a 400-meter track, multiply the number of cones passed by 0.0497 to obtain the distance in miles. For example: if you pass 38 cones on a 440-yard track, 38 x 0.05 = 1.9 miles.

➤ *Interpreting Your Results* Using your recorded scores, consult the charts found in appendixes 4A and 4B to determine your cardiorespiratory fitness level based on this test. Be sure to choose the chart for your sex and age range. Enter the results in your personal fitness results chart (appendix 6).

➤ *Note* Alternatives include walking tests, a treadmill test, a bicycle ergometer test, and a step test. If you have been inactive for many years, it may be advisable to use a walking test rather than the mixed running and walking of the Cooper test. Each of these tests offers advantages and disadvantages, and with proper supervision and monitoring they can be equally effective. Most fitness centers offer supervised fitness testing, and this option may be preferred if you have not been physically active or have any concerns about performing a fitness test.

PUSH-UP TEST

Push-ups demonstrate the muscular fitness of your upper body, including your chest, back, and arms.

➢ **Objective**   Perform the maximum number of push-ups without rest.

➢ **Directions**   Men should perform as many push-ups as possible using standard form and technique and without resting. The body should be supported by hands and toes only. The hands should be placed slightly wider than shoulder-width apart, the feet should be no more than 12 inches (30 centimeters) apart, and the body should be straight from head to heel. Starting with your arms straight, lower your body until your upper arms are parallel to the floor, then return to the starting position. Maintain a straight body from head to heels at all times (see figure 5.2).

Women may do the same or do a modified "bent-knee" push-up. This modified push-up is done by kneeling on the floor, placing your hands on the floor slightly wider than shoulder-width apart, and keeping your back straight throughout the exercise (see figure 5.3).

Count the number of complete push-ups performed, or have a partner count for you. Stop and record your score when you are unable to maintain correct form and technique, have to rest, or simply cannot continue.

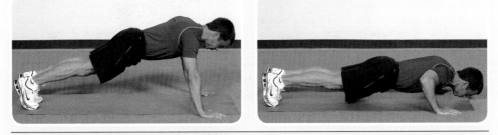

Figure 5.2   Push-up test: standard technique.

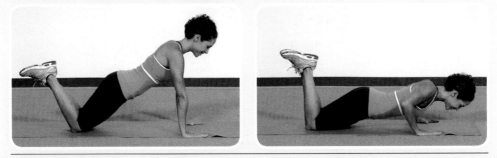

Figure 5.3   Push-up test: modified technique.

➢ **Interpreting Your Results**   Consult the tables in appendixes 2A and 2B to determine your rating on this test. Be sure to select the correct chart for your sex and age group.

SIT-UP TEST

Sit-ups or curl-ups demonstrate the muscular fitness of your abdominals and hip flexors, which are important for core stability and back support.

▷ **Objective**   Perform the maximum number of sit-ups in 1 minute.

▷ **Directions**   We suggest that you find a flat, cushioned surface (e.g., a mat). Lie on your back with your knees bent at approximately a 90-degree angle and your feet flat on the floor and positioned approximately 12 to 18 inches (30 to 45 centimeters) from your buttocks. Have a partner assist you by anchoring your feet to the ground. If no partner is available, you can anchor your feet under a piece of furniture or equipment. Hold your arms flat across your chest with each hand placed on the opposite shoulder. Keeping your arms in position, curl up your trunk and touch your elbows to your knees, then lower yourself until your shoulder blades touch the floor (see figure 5.4). Do not bounce up immediately for the next sit-up; rather, hesitate for 1 second before beginning the next movement. At the end of 1 minute, record your score.

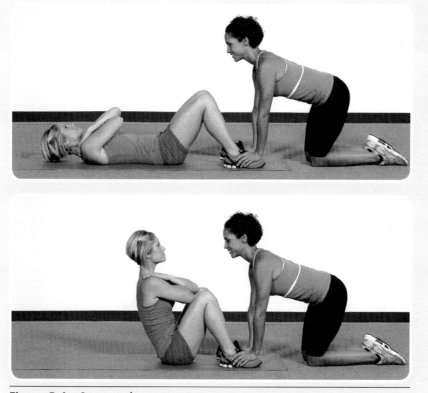

Figure 5.4   Sit-up technique.

▷ **Interpreting Your Results**   Check the charts in appendixes 1A and 1B to determine your rating on this test.

SIT-AND-REACH TEST

The sit-and-reach is a test of flexibility in your lower back, hamstrings, and hips. You will need a yardstick and some tape. Secure the yardstick to the floor by placing a 12-inch (30-centimeter) length of tape across it at the 15-inch (38-centimeter) mark.

➢ **Objective**   Sit and reach forward as far as possible.

➢ **Directions**

1. Warm up for this test by performing gentle to moderate stretching of your entire body, particularly your lower back, hamstrings, and hips. Good choices are the modified hurdler stretch (see page 111 for description) and cat stretch (see page 112).

2. For the test, take a seated position on the floor with the yardstick between your legs (and the zero mark toward you) and the soles of your feet about 12 inches (30 centimeters) apart and exactly even with the tape at the 15-inch (38-centimeter) mark. The test should be performed without shoes.

3. Keeping your legs straight, place one hand on top of the other so that your middle fingers are evenly aligned with each other.

4. Gently lean forward along the yardstick in a slow and controlled manner and reach as far as possible while you exhale. Hold the position for 2 seconds (see figure 5.5). Do not bounce or stretch to the point of pain; either action could produce injury.

5. Note the distance you reached. Then repeat the same movement two more times and choose the best score as the one to record.

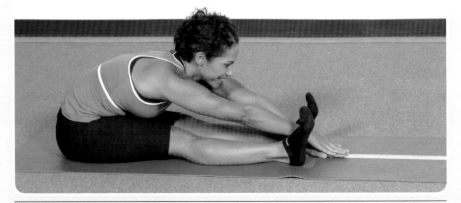

Figure 5.5   Sit-and-reach test.

➢ **Interpreting Your Results**   Check the charts in appendixes 3A and 3B to determine your rating.

BODY COMPOSITION

This test determines the percentage of your body that consists of fat rather than muscle or bone.

In order to ensure accurate results, you need professional assistance with this test. We suggest that you explore the options at commercial gyms, doctors' offices, or health centers. Some professionals in health sciences (e.g., athletic trainers, physical therapists) are also excellent resources.

Of the options available for testing body composition, we prefer that you investigate the possibility of using a Bod Pod, which uses the technique of air displacement. This method is less uncomfortable than underwater weighing, and it is quick and accurate.

Our second choice is bioelectrical impedance analysis (BIA). Once again, the process is comfortable, quick, and convenient. The only drawback has been a relative lack of accuracy as compared with other methods, though we believe that advances in equipment and calculation are ongoing and will improve the reliability of these tests. We would also point out that this equipment is dramatically cheaper to purchase than the equipment for either the water or air displacement methods; therefore, it is more likely to be readily accessible.

In the United States, Bod Pod assessment typically costs about $50. BIA measurement is offered for free at many health, wellness, and fitness centers; check online or make a few calls to determine the options in your community.

Our third choice is to locate a professional who is experienced in using skinfold calipers to measure fat at several locations on the body. This has long been a popular field test for percent body fat because it is readily available and relatively inexpensive. The only issue is reliability across repeated tests, so it is critical that you use an experienced professional and continue to use him or her for repeated tests in order to reduce the chance of error.

USING YOUR FITNESS TEST RESULTS

Don't worry about the results of your fitness tests. Just accept them as important indicators of your current state of fitness and as a starting point for change. In fact, if your results are alarmingly low, you are likely to improve quickly and thus feel great motivation to continue.

You should do a set of identical tests after 4 to 6 weeks of physical activity. It is generally necessary to wait this length of time between tests in order to see significant change.

If your initial scores reveal a more moderate level of fitness, then you are more likely to see rapid improvement, particularly in certain tests, if you choose the right activities to build the fitness you desire. At higher levels of fitness, improvement will come more slowly; in such cases, we assume that your scores reflect the fact that you have been fairly active, and we encourage you to measure your success based on other factors, such as variety, staying free of injury, expanding your exercise experiences, and cross-training.

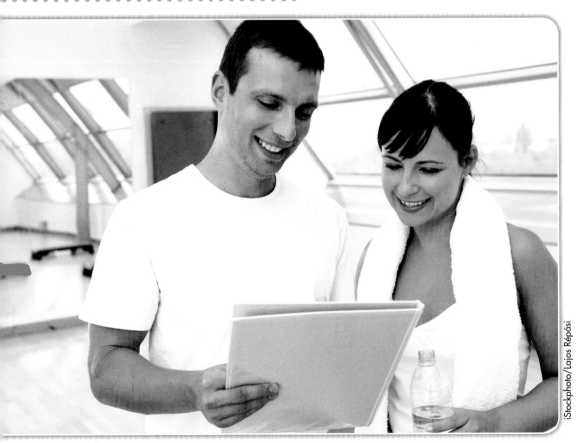

Use your fitness test results as the starting point for change.

The most likely scenario involves variation in scores among tests. Low scores in one area give you a clear message that you need to address that weakness when designing your personal plan for physical activity. If, for example, muscular strength and endurance are areas of weakness, then you'll want to be sure to include a regular routine of strength training in your plan.

Finally, remember that embarking on a more vigorous, sustained program for a lifetime of physical activity means more than just being physically fit at any given point in time. The results of your fitness tests are simply one signpost on a new path to increased physical activity. Our hope is that you explore various options, acquire skills, try new activities, stay injury free, and identify physical activities that you truly enjoy and love to do.

TIPS for High Energy

- Complete the preassessment checklist and consult with your physician before beginning a new program of physical activity.

- Read the instructions for self-testing until you have a clear understanding of each test. Gather the equipment you need, enlist the help of a buddy if possible, or consult a fitness professional who can help you.

- Do not begin the tests until you have properly warmed up your body and performed stretching exercises. This would be a terrible time to injure yourself, just at the beginning of your new effort to be physically active.

- Record the results from your tests in each area and keep them safe but handy so you can use them in developing your personal plan for physical activity.

- Accept the results of the tests objectively and use the information in a helpful way. Don't beat yourself up over past inactivity; you're now on your way to positive change.

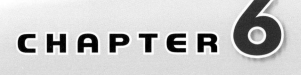

CHAPTER 6

CREATING FUN AND EXHILARATION THROUGH PHYSICAL ACTIVITY

The key to changing your behavior by increasing your level of physical activity is to make it *fun*. It's a lot easier to schedule time for physical activity if you are looking forward to it than if you are feeling like you have a chore to perform. Fun means excitement, pleasure, diversion, recreation, playfulness, and good humor. It creates a mood of well-being that features smiles and laughter. For many people, fun is part and parcel of sports, games, and recreational physical activity. If you have experienced physical activity in the past without the element of fun, is it possible that you chose the wrong sport, game, or workout routine? We think that is likely, and we believe that you can benefit by rethinking your choice of activity.

In this chapter, you'll learn that *fun* means different things to different people; thus part of our goal here is to help you define what can make physical activity fun for *you*. If your past experiences with physical activity have not exactly been fun-filled, then carefully consider our suggestions about what makes activity fun, then test yourself to see whether changing the situation for activity transforms it into an enjoyable experience.

Beyond fun, we look at the phenomenon of exhilaration during and after physical activity. Many athletes report strong feelings of emotional pleasure and increased energy while they are exercising or playing a sport. These feelings may be attributed to one's mind-set during activity, but they are physiologically based and can be attributed to increased secretion of serotonin, which produces a natural high.

The final section in this chapter clarifies the difference between setting performance goals for your physical activity and setting the more common outcome goals. Once you can recognize the difference, you'll enjoy more success, because your achievement of performance goals is totally under your control.

FIGURING OUT WHAT'S FUN FOR YOU

Our experience with thousands of would-be participants in physical activity has led us to believe that it is critical at the outset to examine the various types of fun that can be generated by physical activity. Let's take a look at them and see which ones strike a chord with you.

As you read through the specific categories in the following checklist, assign each one a number between 1 and 5 based on its importance to you (5 for very important, 1 for not important). Completing the list will give you valuable information to use in choosing sports, games, and activities that can be fun for you.

PERSONAL PREFERENCES FOR PHYSICAL ACTIVITY

For each category described in this checklist, write a number between 1 and 5 (5 indicates very important and 1 indicates not important) in the corresponding box to indicate how important that category is to you.

☐ *Venue:* Many people just love certain venues for physical activity, whether because of happy childhood memories, the venue's uniqueness, or perhaps an interest in nature. Where would you prefer to spend time engaged in physical activity? Examine the following list and circle the venues that interest you.

- Indoor facility
- The outdoors
- Fitness gym
- Traditional gym
- Water
- Snow
- Mountains
- Beach
- Golf course
- Tennis court
- Playing field
- Your neighborhood
- Backyard or home gym
- Other: _____

☐ *Physical challenge:* Do you crave physical challenge? Is an element of risk important to you? Do you like to compete against nature, yourself, or other obstacles? Many people enjoy pushing themselves to test their body and their ability to persevere in spite of obstacles or endurance limits. Examples include competing in a marathon, triathlon, or Ironman competition. For some people, the element of risk provides thrills and incentives for engaging in activities such as mountain climbing, mountain biking, and hang gliding.

☐ *Social interaction:* Many of us enjoy physical activity that involves other people. Besides enjoying their company during the activity itself, we often become friends with people we meet through sports or physical activity and choose to spend time with them in other ways as well.

Do you enjoy being part of a team and learning to work and play together as a smoothly functioning unit? Do you look forward to spending time with a group before or after activity in order to just socialize, eat, or drink?

Do you crave meeting new people with similar interests? Are mixed-gender activities of interest to you?

Do you enjoy earning the respect of others for your dedication, effort, attitude, dependability, and teamwork? Is the feeling of belonging to an identifiable group important to you?

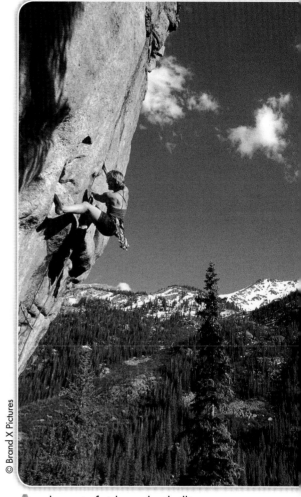

© Brand X Pictures

An element of risk can be thrilling.

Does having an exercise appointment with a friend or friends make it more likely that you'll do everything possible to keep your commitment rather than blow it off? Having this built-in accountability is one of the best ways for many people to ensure that they'll show up every time.

☐ *Family values:* In these days of excessive workloads and busy lives, you may crave more time with your family (most of us do). When you do carve out time for togetherness, do you enjoy doing physical activities together? Consider the physical activities you might share with your spouse, children, or grandchildren. What a pleasure it is to share valuable time doing something that is helpful to all of you! You don't have to be the coach or leader every time. Let your spouse or kids lead the way into a new activity; for example, bicycling, in-line skating, hiking, tennis, and table tennis are great family activities.

(continued)

Personal Preferences   *(continued)*

☐ *Competition:* Many of us grew up competing in sports. Some of us loved it, whereas others despised it. Do you love the thrill of victory, and can you deal with the agony of defeat? When the outcome of a game is on the line, do you smile and embrace the pressure and challenge? Do you like having the tangible evidence of winning to indicate that you're the better team or competitor because of your hard work, skill, strategy, or fitness?

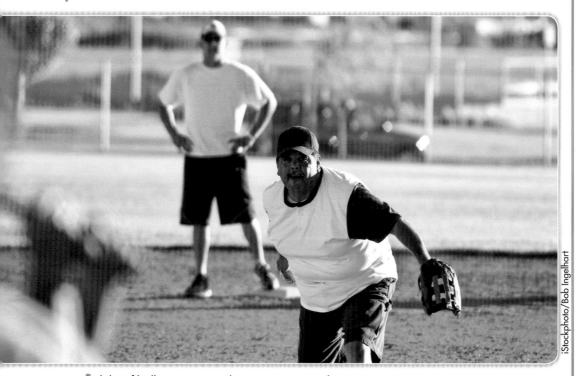

Adult softball teams appeal to team-sport enthusiasts.

☐ *Rewards and recognition:* We are used to receiving rewards for good performance, and some of us have become dependent on them for motivation. Do you enjoy winning medals, trophies, certificates, or other prizes based on your performance? Does seeing your name listed in a newspaper or magazine as a winner or high-ranking performer increase your interest in and commitment to sport or competition?

☐ *Learning new skills:* Learning and practicing new skills can be immensely satisfying. Some people are lifelong lesson takers who just enjoy learning and refining their skills. Are you open to learning new things regardless of age or lack of experience in an activity? Even if you never achieve mastery of a skill, do you simply enjoy learning something new?

☐ *Skill and challenge:* Most athletes report that they enjoy sports most when they achieve a balance between their personal skill and the challenge they undertake (see figure 6.1). If team or personal skills are equal to the challenge, sports can be great fun. On the other hand, a challenge that is too great—for example, competing against an opponent who is overwhelmingly better—can produce anxiety and frustration. Similarly, if your skill far exceeds the challenge, sports can be pretty boring and repetitive. It's not much fun to compete regularly against others when the outcome is clear from the start.

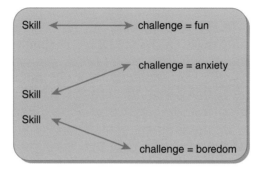

Figure 6.1   What is fun?

Adapted from M.E. Ewing and V. Seefeldt, 1990, American youth and sports participation: A study of 10,000 students and their feelings about sport (North Palm Beach, FL: Athletic Footwear Association).

☐ *Self-confidence and self-efficacy:* These feelings are important to a person's overall concept of self, and they carry over into every part of life. When you participate in physical activity, you have the opportunity to invest energy and effort, mark progress, and achieve goals. The term *self-efficacy* refers to the feeling that your success or failure depends not on others or on luck but on you and the effort you put forth. Most high achievers in any field rely on their own full effort and believe that it will lead to success. People with high self-efficacy typically persevere in spite of obstacles, and the feeling often transfers to other areas of life. Do you already possess high levels of self-confidence and self-efficacy? Could you use physical activity to increase your levels?

☐ *Self-reliance and independence:* Lots of sports and other physical activities offer opportunities for you to perform as an individual. Do you gain satisfaction or relaxation by training or competing by yourself instead of as part of a group? If you find it stressful to think about partners, teammates, and group cohesion, then perhaps it would be a better choice for you to choose an activity that allows you to perform on your own.

☐ *Intellectual challenge and stimulation:* Every physical activity presents its own set of challenges. Sports that involve substantive strategy require clear thinking and good decision making. If you enjoy this type of intellectual challenge, select sports where strategy can be used to overcome physical prowess and where competition is strategic and tactical within a physical framework.

(continued)

Personal Preferences   *(continued)*

☐ *Travel:* Physical activities can be done at home or in your local neighbor-hood, and if you're constrained by time limits then staying close to home may be your best option for now. But if you enjoy travel—either local or at a distance—consider physical activities that require travel or might lead to travel opportunities. Even local competition between teams from different facilities or clubs allows you to see other parts of your home area and meet people you might otherwise never encounter.

Participating in competition elsewhere in your state will take you to new venues and cities and give you a chance to spend time with teammates and competitors away from the distractions of home and work. You might even factor in time to visit with relatives or old friends in the destination city or do some sightseeing during free time.

For those with a bit of wanderlust, a trip to the other side of the country or even overseas may be the ultimate goal. If you are adventurous and curious about the rest of the world, competitive sport could be your ticket to travel. If you live in a cold area, then a trip to engage in a water sport (e.g., surfing, snorkeling) in a warmer climate might become the highlight of your year. If you live in a warmer area, then a trip to the Rockies for a week of snowboarding and skiing might be equally invigorating. Even better, if you can convince yourself to turn off your electronic devices during the day, you might just find that life is sublime!

☐ *Fitness and appearance:* It's fun to feel fit, strong, and confident in your appearance at the same time. If you get comments on your youthful appearance or a new outfit, do you smile, pull back your shoulders, and enjoy the adulation? Some activities will help you achieve these goals more quickly and efficiently than others. For this purpose, a round of golf, for example, does not provide the same benefit offered by a more vigorous sporting activity, a strength training session, or a challenging aerobic run or swim.

To interpret the results, look back over the categories and your ratings. Categories that you rated 4 or 5 seem to resonate with you. They are your keys to having fun through physical activity. Categories that you rated 2 or 3 may hold some promise, especially if you crave variety in activity. Categories that you marked with a 1 are probably not important enough to you to be helpful here.

Now, a few final questions:

• What physical activities are you doing now that involve the categories you rated 4 or 5?

• Which characteristics interest you but are *not* currently addressed in your activity? Make a note of them, and when it comes time to choose new sport activities let them influence your choices.

- Of all the characteristics you picked out, what are the top three in importance for you? Rank them here:

  1. _____

  2. _____

  3. _____

Keep this list handy as you read the next chapter and begin to gather information to help you choose the physical activities that you will include in your personal plan. As you choose sports or activities, be sure that some of them have at least one of the characteristics identified here as being most important to you.

CREATING EXHILARATION

As we explored fun in the previous section, you might have realized that physical activity can be more than fun. Often, it brings on intense feelings of exhilaration. To *exhilarate* means to enliven, make cheerful, stimulate, create passion, and create energy and excitement.

When we think of fun, it may have many levels of intensity, but the term *exhilarate* indicates only extremely high levels of feeling. We have watched two novice tennis players who set a goal of hitting 10 consecutive shots without an error break out in grins or even a giggle as they near their goal. When they exceed their goal, their excitement is undeniable and contagious. Similarly, picture the triumphant arms-raised gesture of any soccer player who scores a goal. Why not strive for such feelings of exhilaration during and after *your* physical activity?

Let's take a closer look at the possible psychological benefits of physical activity on mood, feelings, and mental health. It has been well documented that exercise and physical activity can have positive effects on your psychological well-being in both the short and long terms. Physical activity helps reduce anxiety and depression. Simply engaging in exercise has a therapeutic effect and helps counter unpleasant emotions, and the type and intensity of exercise affect the benefit you receive.

Generally, research has shown that you can lower anxiety by engaging in aerobic exercise—continuous physical activity during which oxygen is transported to the working muscles to allow you to continue activity—for a duration of 30 to 60 minutes with a heart rate of at least 70 percent of your maximum. Examples are brisk walking, running, jogging, cycling, swimming, aerobics, rowing, and cross-country skiing. Muscle tension is similarly decreased. You might note that if the duration or intensity is lowered below the recommended 70 percent, the effect on anxiety is minimal.

This pattern holds if you exercise on a regular basis—say, three to five times a week. The frequency of exercise is important because the benefits of physical activity on anxiety generally wear off after about 24 hours. For those who

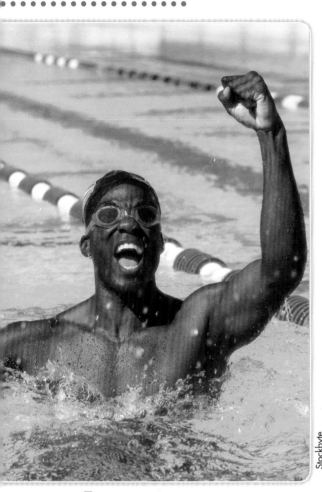

Exhilaration!

Stockbyte

suffer from depression, the intensity of exercise is not as critical as the frequency; in fact, a moderate level of activity appears to be best.

Mood changes, which we all experience, clearly occur after exercise. Feelings of happiness, elation, and well-being often last for a day or even several days after activity. Such feelings have been noted in runners so often that the phenomenon has been called the runner's high, which refers to a euphoric sensation of arousal, a heightened awareness of surroundings, and a feeling of transcending time and space. Many of us have experienced such feelings after vigorous activity in a sport, game, or workout.

Some have theorized that physical activity also provides a distraction from other areas of life. While engaged in vigorous activity, most of us simply can't exert energy on worrying or thinking about problems, issues, or concerns. Thus exercise reduces our stress by distracting us, at least for the moment, and helps steady our emotions and mood (Weinberg and Gould 2007).

Finally, we know that physical activity brings on various physiological changes that affect our mood. During exercise, our brain and various organs (e.g., the pituitary and adrenal glands) secrete endorphins, which reduce sensations of pain and may produce a state of euphoria. Recent research has also shown that physical activity can have a powerful effect on generating new cells in the brain and strengthening the network of neural connections between cells. In fact, research in education has shown remarkable improvement in students' ability to tackle tough problems in math and science immediately following a period of physical activity (Ratey 2008).

Thus, physical activity can be not only fun but also exhilarating! To be sure, this effect is not automatic. You need to choose your sport or activity wisely in order to enjoy the intensely positive feelings that are possible.

Before we leave this section, we invite you to do a little self-assessment. The point of this exercise is to help you identify experiences that have produced exhilaration for you either during or after physical activity—and plan to re-create them. If it turns out that you've never created such feelings, you may want to give it a try now that you have a better understanding of why and how they are likely to occur. Consider the following questions:

- Have you ever felt euphoria like that of a runner's high after intense physical activity?
  - If so, try to re-create that experience in your mind and describe how you believe you achieved it.
  - If you have never experienced such a feeling, do you attribute this to a lack of intensity or duration in your typical exercise routine?
- What activities that interest you are most likely to increase your chances of experiencing such feelings? (Remember, activities most likely to produce exhilaration are aerobic, moderately or highly intense, and at least 30 minutes long.) Make a note here of those activities:

  1. _____

  2. _____

  3. _____

MAKING PHYSICAL ACTIVITY FUN

Some of you may be thinking that your own experiences with physical activity haven't been much fun and that they certainly have not produced good feelings afterward. We know that is a possibility, and we wonder if you might benefit from adjusting your approach. Let's look at some likely causes. Have you ever had these thoughts after engaging in physical activity?

- Wow, that was brutal! I sure don't ever want to punish myself like that again.
- After this workout, I'll need at least a week to recover.
- I'm exhausted. Looks like I'll be spending the rest of the day on the couch.
- My body hurts all over. I can't even smile, but I guess I'll get over it in a few days.
- I'm afraid I'm injured, but it's the weekend and I don't even know where to get help. I hope my injury [e.g., back, foot, knee, hamstring] isn't serious. Guess I'll just rest it and lay off for a while.
- Boring! I'm getting tired of the same old routine. It seemed fun for a while, but the novelty has worn off.

If any of these thoughts has occurred to you, you are not alone. The more inactive you have been, the more likely it is that you'll feel this way at first.

Most of us experience this type of thinking on occasion, but if it happens to you on a regular basis, then some changes are in order as you make your plan for physical activity. Here are a few modifications to consider that might put a smile back on your face and make your physical activity fun:

- Know your limits! When you begin to feel ill or at risk for injury, stop your physical activity gradually and allow your body to recover for at least 24 hours. You may be able to push through the first onset of pain or discomfort, but if it reoccurs, listen to your body.

- Be sure to allot 10 to 15 minutes for cool-down activity after exercise to allow your muscles to recover naturally; use static stretches during this time. If you adhere to this routine, you'll reduce your muscle stiffness and soreness after activity.

- Vary your activities so that you cross-train all your muscles. Integrating various activities helps prevent overuse injuries of specific body parts. Not only will your body be happier, but your mind will enjoy the change as well.

- Absolutely factor in some rest and recovery days, especially after hard workouts. If you have a particularly vigorous day, follow it with light movement, stretching, or perhaps a leisurely swim or walk.

- Seek out new partners, opponents, or venues to keep your activity fresh and interesting. Even just shifting a run from the track to the beach or a park offers a great variation.

- Vary your pattern over the years by trying new activities, trying a new facility, seeking out new exercise partners (including your significant other), or adjusting to the seasons of the year. Repeating the same old pattern often results in boredom and drudgery. Be creative, innovative, and open to new experiences.

USING PERFORMANCE GOALS TO CREATE FUN, SUCCESS, AND SATISFACTION

We encourage you to create performance goals (sometimes called mastery goals) to ensure that you'll have fun and be more satisfied with the results of your physical activity. The only requirement for achieving a performance goal is that you make a full commitment to investing energy and effort toward achieving it. The genius of this type of goal, then, is that you can fully control your progress toward it, which of course greatly increase your chance of success. People who are high achievers tend to adopt performance goals, thus taking full personal responsibility for their eventual success or failure.

In contrast, some people have been conditioned to evaluate their success in terms of outcome goals. Such goals are often expressed in terms of winning a

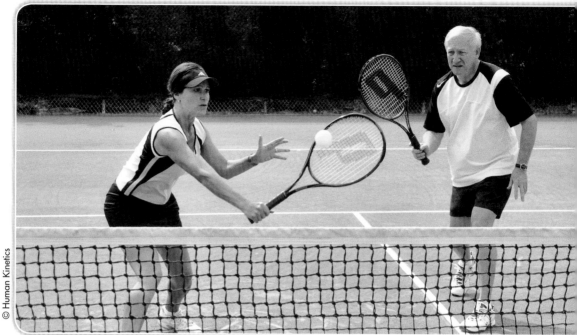

© Human Kinetics

Tennis is the fastest-growing traditional sport in America, up 43 percent since the year 2000 according to the Sporting Goods Manufacturers Association (SGMA).

game, setting a record, achieving a personal best, or conquering nature in some manner. Regrettably, such goals are not fully under your control; they can be affected by your opponent, the weather, or another environmental condition. Most low achievers attribute their failure to their low ability or skill, which only sets them up for subsequent failures as a self-fulfilling prophecy.

The earlier discussion of making physical activity fun implied that success or competency leads to feelings of fun so long as the challenge is appropriate for your skill or ability. Since you are much more likely to succeed in achieving performance or mastery goals than outcome goals, we can promise that you will have more fun in your physical activities if you craft some performance goals such as those listed below.

- Each time I play, I will practice my tennis serve by hitting 25 serves into the target area before I leave the court.
- Before I exercise, I will take a full 10 minutes to warm up and stretch (using dynamic stretches) before beginning the activity. I will also give myself time to cool down and stretch before ending the session.
- Before I play a round of golf, I will spend 10 minutes warming up by using dynamic movements similar to those I use in my golf swing. I will then go to the practice range for at least a half dozen shots with each

club I expect to use that day. Finally, after a dozen practice putts on the putting green, I will be fully prepared to play.

- When weather conditions are unfavorable, I will complete my workout and resist the temptation to cut it short or eliminate it altogether.

Note that each of these goals requires only that you adopt it and expend effort and energy toward achieving it. No one else can affect the outcome. In contrast, here are some typical outcome goals:

- We're going to win the game on Saturday and go to the league championship.
- My goal is to finish first in each race I enter in the master's division.
- I plan to reach the top of the mountain no matter what nature sends my way.
- Our goal is to win the club championship this year.
- My goal for today is to finish in the top three.

Notice that achievement of these outcome goals depends on the level of competition, the performance of opponents, and even nature itself. You simply can't control these factors, and you may well resort to blaming a poor result on bad luck or on a lack of talent on your part.

We recommend that you practice writing performance (mastery) goals once you've decided which activities you'd like to pursue. We revisit this topic in chapter 8, which helps you develop your personal exercise prescription.

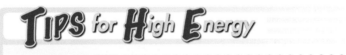

- Aim to have fun during physical activity.
- Choose several categories of fun from the list in this chapter and be sure they are reflected in your activity plan.
- Don't overlook the opportunity to generate exhilaration through sports and physical activity. Experiment with various activities until you find several that help you achieve the physical and psychological state of euphoria that you'll never forget.
- Learn to set reasonable performance (mastery) goals for physical activities so that you have a realistic chance of success.
- If physical activity is not fun for you, then change your routine, the venue, your workout partners, or the activity itself.
- Factor in rest days for recovery; learn your limits and listen to your body.

CHAPTER 7

GATHERING INFORMATION

To develop a personal prescription for physical activity (the topic of chapter 8), you first have to spend some time and effort gathering information about possible choices. Most books or programs for physical fitness advocate increasing your level of physical activity through daily physical endeavors such as walking, climbing stairs, or working around the house or garden. Others send you directly to the fitness gym to use expensive equipment for aerobic work or strength training.

Our approach is broader. We want you to seriously consider a wide range of physical activities to get you started and keep you on the path to more exercise. At the heart of our approach is the idea of making physical activity into something fun and even exhilarating rather than just another daily commitment like going to work. By opening yourself up to a wide range of activities, you ensure variety in your options and give yourself the opportunity to change activities when forced to by relocation, weather, loss of income, injury, or simple boredom. We also firmly believe that in participating in a range of activities, you will be doing your body a big favor by reducing your risk for typical overuse injuries. Even sports or physical activities that generally provide excellent exercise can cause problems if performed too often at high intensity or without adequate rest and recovery time.

This chapter leads you through the steps for considering a wide range of physical activities that you might want to pursue. Once you have established your interest in certain sports or activities, the next step is to match them with the fitness components you want to develop: cardiorespiratory fitness, muscular fitness, flexibility, and good body composition. You will benefit from ensuring that each of these components is covered in the final personal prescription for activity that you develop in chapter 8. In order to address all four components, you will likely need to include a number of different activities.

Another item of business for this chapter is to consider your activity choices in terms of the fun factor discussed in chapter 6. If an activity is not likely to rate high on your personal scale for fun, then it is doubtful that you'll sustain it over the long term. We also encourage you to research your local community in order to locate facilities for physical activity, identify groups that promote or conduct activities in which you are interested, and determine the approximate cost of participation.

Finally, if you are relatively new to a sport or activity, we help you decide whether it is wise to seek professional instruction from the outset. Choosing a coach or instructor can be confusing, but it may also be crucial to your long-term success.

CHOOSING SPORTS AND PHYSICAL ACTIVITIES

This section helps you organize your research by presenting a list of physical activity choices as a starting point. To help you organize your analysis, the list is divided into 10 categories. Once you have identified appealing options, you will then need to consider their availability in your area by assessing factors such as weather, natural environment, organizations, public facilities, commercial facilities, and cost.

We also try to help you avoid limiting your choices due to lack of information about alternative ways to perform various physical activities to achieve your goals. There may be a way for you to participate in an attractive option even if the solution is not readily apparent or traditional for that sport or activity.

Finally, we ask you to consider how the activity options discussed in this chapter match up with the definitions of fun that you rated highly in chapter 6. It makes sense to choose sports or physical activities that are most likely to meet your personal needs for fun and enjoyment so that your motivational level remains high.

Begin gathering information by reviewing the sports and physical activities listed in figure 7.1 and making notes to yourself about how the activities of interest to you might fit into your personal prescription.

Step 1   Choose the physical activities that hold some interest for you right now and make a note of them in the first column of figure 7.2.

Step 2   For each activity you choose, write an *R, C,* or *F* in the second column of figure 7.2 to indicate whether it interests you as a recreational, competitive, or fitness endeavor.

- *Recreational* activities are social, relaxing, and enjoyable; they involve little or no competition.
- *Competitive* activities or sports involve some level of competition against others.
- *Fitness* activities are oriented toward physical movement that enhances your physical fitness.

FIGURE 7.1 SPORT AND PHYSICAL ACTIVITY CHECKLIST

Fitness Activities
Aerobics (high, low, or step)
Boot camp workouts
Calisthenics or exercise with music
Cardio kickboxing
Elliptical machine work
Fitness running
Fitness swimming
Fitness walking
Pilates
Rowing machine work
Spinning (stationary cycling classes)
Stair climbing
Stretching
Tai chi
Treadmill walking or running
Yoga

Other Aerobic Activities
Biking
In-line skating
Interval training
Jogging
Running
Swimming
Walking

Strength Training
Body weight
Exercise ball
Free weights
Medicine balls
Resistance bands
Resistance machines

Team Sports
Basketball
Football (touch or flag)
Ice hockey
Lacrosse
Rugby
Soccer
Softball
Street hockey
Ultimate (Frisbee)
Volleyball

Individual Sports
Cross-country running
Marathon or minimarathon
Track and field
Triathlon

Racket and Skill Sports
Badminton
Bowling
Golf
Handball
Racquetball
Squash
Table tennis
Tennis

Outdoor Activities
Adventure racing
Archery
Climbing (mountain or rock)
Hiking
Horseback riding
Mountain biking
Orienteering
Paintball

Winter Sports
Ice skating
Skiing (downhill or cross-country)
Snowboarding

Water Sports
Canoeing
Kayaking
Rowing
Sailing
Scuba diving
Snorkeling
Surfing
Water skiing

Dance
Ballet, tap, and modern
Ballroom
Competitive
Folk or ethnic
Latin
Social
Square

| FIGURE 7.2 | My Sport and Activity Choices |

Activity	Type of activity (R,C,F)	Social? (S)	Limitations?	Experience, skill, knowledge	Fitness component(s) affected	Fun?
1.						
2.						
3.						
4.						
5.						
6.						
7.						
8.						
9.						
10.						
11.						
12.						

From R. Woods and C. Jordan with the Human Performance Institute, 2010, *Energy every day* (Champaign, IL: Human Kinetics).

Step 3   In the third column, make a check mark for your chosen activities that involve a social component.

Step 4   If you anticipate any limitations (e.g., seasonal, scheduling) that could affect your chosen activities, note this information in the fourth column.

Step 5   Evaluate your own experience, skill, and knowledge in each activity you've chosen. In column 5, rate each activity choice from 1 (least) to 5 (most).

Step 6   Now review your list and eliminate any activities for which you may have a disqualifying physical or psychological limitation—for example, physical injury or weakness, effects of aging, fear of heights, or lack of eye–hand coordination.

Step 7   Review your final selections and project whether each activity will affect you in the following areas:

a. Cardiorespiratory fitness

b. Muscular strength and endurance

c. Flexibility

d. Body composition

Write an *a*, *b*, *c*, or *d* beside each activity (in the sixth column) to indicate which of these four components of your health will be affected by that activity. If you find that, taken together, your choices do not address all four components of fitness, review the activity list and add a few activities to cover any remaining components.

Step 8   Using your selected activity list as it now looks, estimate how much fun each activity is likely to be based on your own experience or current feelings (5 for great fun, 1 for not very fun). After taking this step, your working list should look like the sample shown in figure 7.3.

FIGURE 7.3	**Sample Completed Sport and Activity Choices**					
Activity	Type of activity (R,C,F)	Social? (S)	Limitations?	Experience, skill, knowledge	Fitness component(s) affected	Fun?
1. *Walking*	R	S		5	a, b, d	3
2. *Yoga*	F		Classes	1	b, c	2
3. *Swimming*	R, F		Weather	3	a, c, d	5
4. *Interval training*	F			4	a, b, d	3
5. *Free weights*	F	S	Time	5	b, d	4
6. *Soccer*	R	S	Team to join	1	a, d	5
7. *Tennis*	R, F	S	Time	2	a, d	4
8. *Stretching*	F		Motivation	1	c	1
9. *Mountain biking*	R, F	S	Geography	2	a, b	4
10. *Snowboarding*	R	S	Geography, cost	2	a, b	4
11. *Sprinting*	C		Local events	1		4
12. *Pilates*	F		Classes	2	b, c	3

You will probably need to eliminate some activities because they are not available or are available only during part of the year due to weather or sporting seasons. You also may find that some activities are simply out of your price range. It is our hope, however, that you will conclude that at least half of your chosen activities can remain on your list so that you have some variety of choice, both now and in the future.

ASSESSING LOCAL PHYSICAL ACTIVITY OPPORTUNITIES

Now that you have chosen a list of sports and physical activities to explore, you need to do a little digging to see what is available in your neighborhood. Potential resources include your own home as well as activity- and sport-specific groups and private and commercial facilities.

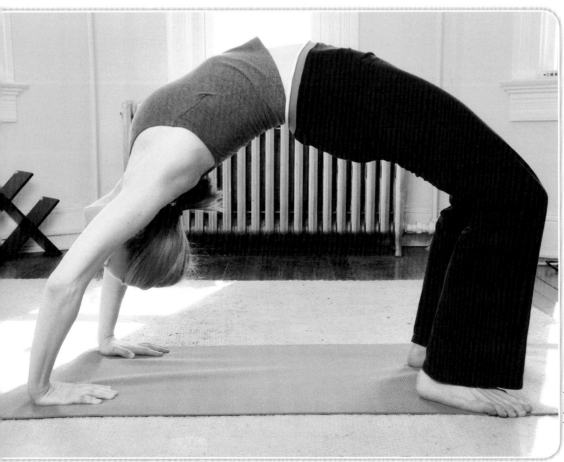

iStockphoto/Nancy Honeycutt

▲ home workout space is convenient, affordable, and involves no travel time.

Your Home

The first question to answer is whether your own home might serve as a venue or launching pad for at least some of your physical activities. The very real advantages of your home are that it is easily accessible, affordable, and involves no travel time. You may already have (or be able to purchase and maintain) suitable equipment for walking, running, strength training, flexibility activity, skating, Pilates, exercise with music, swimming, biking, table tennis, dancing, or working with fitness machines.

If you have a clean, pleasant workout room or area in your home, you might need only to equip it with some relatively inexpensive equipment to begin: exercise ball, dumbbell weights, resistance bands, exercise mat, jump rope, music system, television for exercise videos, and mirrors to check that you are performing movements correctly. Later on, as your budget permits, you might add other equipment for variety and new challenges.

Sport- or Activity-Specific Groups

If some of your sports and physical activities involve groups, you will need to find out when and where people gather. Check out local organizations devoted to the particular activity, contact them, and gather as much information as you can. Many groups have age requirements, limits on size of group, or costs associated with joining that may eliminate them from your list at this time.

A great alternative is to investigate publicly financed programs offered through your local department of recreation. Public facilities throughout the United States offer team or group activities free of charge or at modest cost. You might also check with the local school district or community college about relevant adult education courses. Many schools and colleges open their facilities (fields, tennis courts, basketball courts, swimming pools) to the public at certain times as part of their service to community taxpayers.

Other community agencies offering programs for sport and physical activity include churches (especially basketball and softball leagues), YMCAs and YWCAs, and Jewish community centers. These agencies typically receive some public support and therefore offer affordable rates for recreation and good healthy activities.

Even if your sport or activity does not require a group, it might make sense to join one. For example, introductory golf, tennis, Pilates, yoga, or swimming lessons are typically more fun when done as part of a group. This approach also tends to be less expensive and, perhaps most important, can introduce you to others who are at the same stage of learning and who might become activity buddies for you.

Private and Commercial Facilities

If you are able to afford the cost, many private or commercial facilities offer excellent sports programs and other physical activities. Their facilities are often

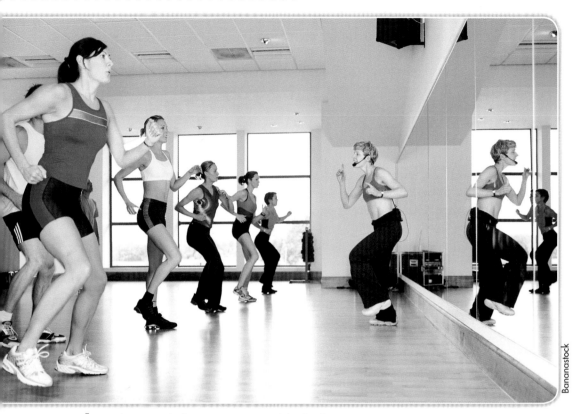

Bananastock

Join other people for activity at a public facility.

of high quality in order to attract a discriminating client base, and those who join are usually very committed to using the facilities. In fact, for many people the added expense increases their motivation to actually use the facility!

One facility category that is often overlooked includes resorts and hotels in your area. They probably built their facilities as an amenity for guests, only to find out that they are underused at certain times of the day or year. Thus you may be able to gain access to a top-of-the-line facility during off-peak hours or days for a very reasonable fee. The most common facilities in these settings are fitness gyms, workout rooms, swimming pools, tennis courts, and golf courses. You might also want to investigate the spa or periodically get a massage.

If you seek higher skill levels in an activity, more competition, or a strong social component, then some sort of private or commercial facility may be your best bet. After all, you can play tennis at the local high school courts for free, but you will likely not have a teaching professional there to provide instruction or organize programs and playing partners. There will also be little social interaction and no special events at the high school courts, and the facilities or environment may be less appealing or out of date. Here's where you need to decide what level of financial commitment you can and want to make.

Informational Resources

Finding organized groups and facilities might require a little digging. To find out what is available in your area, we suggest that you consult four main sources:

- You can find ample information on the Internet by looking up any sport or activity in your area. You can also look into local recreational programs, adult continuing education offerings, commercial facilities open to the public, and private facilities. Many of these groups maintain Web sites that provide you with a wealth of information and choices.

- The yellow pages of your phone book can also be helpful. They provide limited information about programs, facilities, and organizations, but once you gather basic information from the yellow pages, you can find more details through an online search.

- Local libraries often hold a variety of publications that can provide you with information about organizations and facilities. Ask your local librarian for help so that you don't waste time looking in the wrong places.

- People in your community, including friends, often know about physical activities through their own experiences or through word of mouth. Neighbors, work colleagues, social acquaintances, church members, and social clubs can serve as a gold mine of information. As you begin to make contacts to gather information, ask the person you're speaking with about alternatives and options.

As you gather information, be sure to ask about the cost of joining a team, program, or facility. Find out the estimated monthly expense and compare it with your ability to pay. You may find that some sports, programs, or clubs are simply out of your price range. However, don't automatically rule out a sport or physical activity on the basis of cost, because there is probably a less expensive way to participate. For example, using public golf and tennis courts is considerably less expensive than joining a private club, and it may suit your purposes just fine.

COACHING AND INSTRUCTION

If you are interested in trying a new sport or physical activity, we hope you'll consider seeking out professional guidance in the early stages. An experienced coach can help you grasp the fundamental skills and strategies at the outset, thus speeding up your learning experience.

Instead of depending on the unreliable trial-and-error learning method, which may never lead you to the proper technique or strategy, it makes good sense to begin with expert instruction. You'll have more fun participating if you make steady progress right from the start, and you'll be safer too. In fact, some activities almost demand expert instruction because they contain an element of physical risk. Examples include scuba diving, snorkeling, horseback riding, shooting, surfing, rock climbing, hiking, and various fitness activities. In addition, some sports require a certain degree of skill development in order to reach a level of proficiency that is enjoyable. Examples include skiing, snowboarding, dancing, tennis, golf, volleyball, squash, racquetball, and handball.

To search for a suitable instructor, we suggest that you follow a few guidelines. First, most sports activities have at least some certification process for coaching, and you should choose a coach who has demonstrated a level of proficiency attested to by an outside body. If you are unsure, contact the sport's governing body for assistance. For a list of national governing bodies, check the Web site for the U.S. Olympic Committee at www.usoc.org. If the national governing body for a given sport does not certify coaches, it can refer you to organizations that do. Fitness instructors are usually certified by the National Strength and Conditioning Association or by the American College of Sports Medicine. Additionally, many fitness instructors hold college degrees in a related field, such as exercise physiology, kinesiology, or athletic training.

Second, determine the coach's experience in teaching beginners. It doesn't matter how many state or national champions a coach has produced if you are at a beginning level. What matters is whether she or he has successfully introduced people to the sport or activity (and whether those students are still active in it). Third, ask friends and acquaintances for local references just as you would in choosing a doctor, dentist, or chiropractor. Inquire about personality, patience with new learners, teaching style, professionalism, availability, and other issues of importance to you.

Don't be fooled by former athletes or weightlifters who may now be offering their services as teachers. There is little correlation between elite performance and success at teaching beginners in any activity; in fact, some former top athletes demonstrate little empathy for beginners. What matters is to find a coach or instructor who is passionate about helping you improve your skill and who has the teaching skills and patience to help you learn. You'll be able to judge that after one or two trial sessions.

It can also be extremely helpful to find a personal mentor in your sport or activity of choice, either instead of or in addition to a coach. Though mentors are not professionals, you may find an enthusiastic person who has years of firsthand experience and is willing to patiently share that knowledge with you. Most people who truly love their chosen activities are eager to share their passion with others, and they can help you avoid the silly mistakes they have made in the past. In return, you might trade for their time with a free dinner or some service you can provide to show your appreciation.

You might also consider whether to join a learning group for people at the same level in your chosen activity or seek private instruction. Our bias is toward groups for the following reasons. First, you'll meet new people who may become playing partners and friends. In addition, cost is reduced since you all help pay the instructor's fee, and you gain confidence from seeing that others sometimes struggle just as you do. However, one caution we'd share is that no matter the size of the group, all of you should be busy and actively learning during the entire time. A skilled group instructor knows how to structure the learning environment just like a school teacher does. A poor teacher simply instructs one person at a time while others wait their turn. Imagine having to learn to read or do math in that way. Some people prefer to pay for private instruction because their style of learning demands individual attention or because they lack confidence to perform in a group. If you identify with those characteristics and are able and willing to pay, then do what is right for you.

Our best advice is that, if possible, you at least give coaching or group instruction a try, especially in the early stages of learning a new sport or activity. We think you'll have more fun, learn more quickly, and meet new people with the same interest. You'll also have at least one more person who is invested in your success and continuation in the chosen activity. If you miss a class, chances are that you'll get a call reminding you about your commitment and prompting you to schedule your next session.

THE FUN FACTOR

Now that you have developed your own working list of sports and physical activities, go back to chapter 6 to review the section on the various definitions of fun. Evaluate your list of activities in this light and see if you can anticipate why the activities you have chosen might be fun for you. Is it because you like to learn new skills, compete, be outside, or enjoy social camaraderie? Make a note beside each of your chosen sports and physical activities that describes why you expect it to be fun.

Consider also whether it is possible that, with modifications in your approach, the same activity could change from fun to not so fun. If so, how? For example, say that you've chosen your home workout space for stretching, yoga, and strength training. Since you already have the knowledge and skill, you believe your home base is the most convenient and least expensive choice. In thinking further, however, you realize that one reason you enjoyed these activities in the past was learning new routines and skills and sharing the experience with a group. If they were important factors to you then, perhaps you will be disappointed with performing the

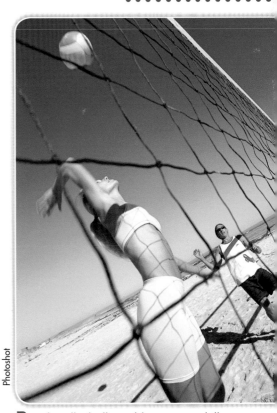

Photoshot

Beach volleyball is a blast at any skill level.

same routines by yourself at home. Be careful about choices like these—that is, ones that have an identifiable possibility of disappointing you.

Consider another example, this one involving swimming. Say that you have fond childhood memories of spending hours around a pool and, indeed, that you became quite a good swimmer. Now, you decide to join a masters athlete competitive program for adults over age 50. Your goal is to improve your times in specific events sufficiently to qualify for the state games for senior athletes. However, if you have never trained for competitive swimming before, you may be surprised by the discipline required to repeatedly swim laps in order to whip yourself into competitive shape. You may decide that you feel more comfortable joining a more recreational swim club or one that combines swimming with cycling and running.

After collecting information, you should be able to establish reasonable priorities about which activities and facilities are good choices for you. We hope that you've come up with at least a half dozen or more, so that you have enough options to make this seem like a fun adventure. Equipped with this information, you're now ready to start creating your personal plan for physical activity.

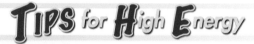

Tips for High Energy

- Using our checklist of sports and activities, identify the ones that are of interest to you. If you can add any others that we have overlooked, please do so.
- Develop a list of your personal choices and, using the codes discussed in this chapter, note the characteristics of each of your choices in figure 7.2.
- Now begin to research the opportunities in your community by using the Internet, the phone book, libraries, and friends and acquaintances. Consider facilities, sponsoring organizations, and costs of programs or memberships.
- Don't forget to compare your list with the fun factors you rated in chapter 6.
- If you are new to a given physical activity, consider getting some coaching or other instruction at the start.

CHAPTER 8

DEVELOPING YOUR PERSONAL PRESCRIPTION FOR PHYSICAL ACTIVITY

I t is finally time to put your personal prescription on paper. We think you'll particularly enjoy this chapter, since it focuses on putting to use all the thinking, research, and analysis you've done during your reading of the preceding chapters. Using the information you have collected—the assessment tests, the fun factor checklist, your sport and activity preferences, and research into the activity programs and facilities available in your local community—your next step is to prepare your plan for using physical activity to pump up your energy.

We don't expect this to be a final long-term plan, since modifications are bound to be needed along the way. At the very least, however, you should now be able to put together a logical plan that appeals to you, is based on sound information, is affordable, and will improve your level of physical fitness. And you should be able to have fun while doing your chosen physical activities or sports.

This is the time for you to choose a number of sports or physical activities to make up your personal exercise prescription. Once you've made your choices, we ask you to consider them in light of your fitness testing results from chapter 5 to determine whether they address your fitness needs. Then we ask you to map out a plan for the frequency, duration, and intensity of each activity to ensure that your plan can produce the changes you desire. The ultimate goal for this chapter is for you to choose several physical activities or sports in which to participate during the next 2 weeks. At that point, you should be ready to make any needed adjustments or realize that it makes sense to simply continue along the same path.

CHOOSING YOUR FIRST ACTIVITIES

It's time now to begin fashioning your personal prescription. Start by looking at the list of sports and physical activities you have chosen to consider. Which ones should you start with? Let's look at some factors that can guide your choices. First, evaluate the sports or physical activities you've selected in light of the four components of fitness described in chapter 7:

- Cardiorespiratory fitness
- Muscular strength and endurance
- Flexibility
- Body composition

Refer back to your notes in figure 7.2, where you marked which of the four fitness components each of your chosen activities and sports is likely to affect. This information may help you determine which choices are most critical to achieving your personal fitness goals.

Next, refer to your fitness test results, which you recorded in appendix 6. If you were particularly weak in a given area, be sure that it is addressed by the activities and sports you choose now for your personal prescription for physical activity. For example, if your flexibility was below average, be sure to include flexibility training and stretching in your prescription. If your aerobic capacity was below average, we suggest that you include walking in your initial prescription. You know how to walk, it is easy to do so either outdoors or indoors (on a treadmill or at a shopping mall), and your risk of injury is minimal. You can also progress easily from a modest workout to a more strenuous one in a matter of a few weeks by increasing the intensity or duration of your walking.

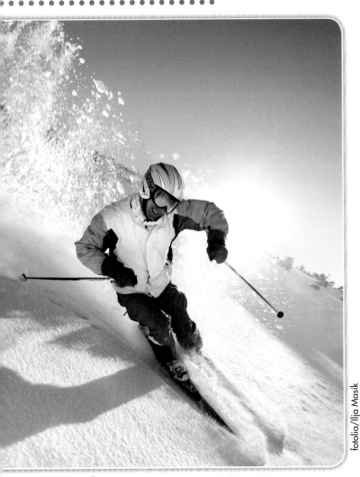

fotolia/Ilja Masik

A blend of excitement, skill, and fun.

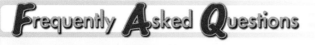

Frequently Asked Questions

Q: What if I haven't done anything physical for several years?

A: Start with a walking program for cardiorespiratory fitness, learn some proper flexibility training exercises, and use your body weight or resistance bands to develop muscular strength and endurance. Each of these activities is easily done and will help you get moving again. But even here, make sure to include the fun factor. You might also pick one sport or activity to learn about and build some skill in—for example, a beginning class in Pilates, yoga, tennis, golf, or scuba diving. You need to have at least one activity that you regularly look forward to with keen anticipation.

Next, pick the physical activity or sport that looks like the most fun to you. Include it in your prescription to add zest, excitement, and perhaps even exhilaration to your activities. We predict that if you leave out fun, your activity program won't last long!

DETERMINING TIME AND EFFORT

Once you've settled on the sports and activities you will start with, it is time to determine how often you will do them, for how long, and at what intensity. The key words here are *frequency, duration,* and *intensity.*

- Frequency is the number of times per week that you perform an activity.
- Duration is the length of time you are active each time you do the activity.
- Intensity is the amount of effort or energy you expend, as measured by your heart rate, by perceived (subjective) exertion, or by weight lifted.

These concerns are critical to ensuring that your program enables you to make fitness improvements. For each criterion (frequency, duration, and intensity), certain minimum requirements have been established on the basis of nationally accepted standards supported by research.

In general, the more you do in terms of each criterion, the greater your fitness improvements will be. It is important, however, to start any activity at a level that is appropriate for you. If you have not been physically active for 6 months or more, start with the minimum requirements and increase your effort gradually. The worst mistake you can make is to set overly ambitious goals that produce extreme stiffness or soreness or even an overuse injury that forces you to stop the activity before you really get into a routine. Mild muscle soreness is to be expected, but if soreness becomes severe you are more likely to withdraw due to the pain. While many athletes have adhered to the adage "No pain, no gain" in their training, we do not recommend that approach, particularly if you have been inactive for some time.

If, on the other hand, you have been following a regular physical activity program for 6 months or more, then consider increasing the frequency, duration, or intensity. The key word here is *progression.* Start easy, then gradually build your physical activity program.

Finally, regardless of which physical activities you choose, they must fit into your schedule. Don't plan to do something every Monday, Wednesday, and Friday evening if that is not practical or realistic. If you do, your program will not last. We recommend that you decide on an appropriate starting frequency, duration, and intensity and stick to this formula for 2 weeks before you adjust the levels.

Frequency and Duration

Here are some general guidelines for determining frequency and duration (Centers for Disease Control and Prevention 2008). We look first at aerobic training, then at strength and flexibility work.

• Generally, you should perform a weekly total of 150 minutes of moderately intense aerobic activity such as brisk walking. For example, you could do 30 minutes of activity on 5 days each week.

Remember, however, that something is better than nothing, and even doing 10 minutes at a time can be helpful. If you have difficulty scheduling 30-minute blocks, try going for a brisk 10-minute walk three times a day, five times a week. You could walk once before work, once at lunchtime, and once after work. This pattern would give you a total of 150 minutes of moderately intense aerobic activity each week.

Remember, too, that any continuous movement can be aerobic in nature and that even short bursts of activity throughout your day may increase your fitness. Indeed, you may be surprised at how much activity you can accumulate each week simply by making the most of movement opportunities. For example, always take the stairs instead of the elevator, park farther away from your office to increase your walk to the building, take a walking break at midmorning and midafternoon (this will boost your energy as well!), go shopping (and walk around a mall for a couple of hours), or play outdoors with your children or grandchildren.

Generally, the more you do (in terms of frequency, duration, and intensity), the greater benefits you receive. As we mentioned earlier, however, progression is the key. Start easy and gradually increase your activity; even elite athletes can injure themselves by doing too much. In fact, as you progress in your fitness activity, you should consider the fact that you can get even greater health benefits by accumulating 300 minutes of moderately intense aerobic activity during each week—for example, 60 minutes of brisk walking on 5 days per week.

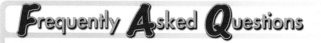

Q: My personal schedule is so busy that I just can't seem to find time to devote 60 minutes to physical activity. I find that changing clothes, driving to the field or gym, and showering afterward add on another half hour. An hour and a half out of my day is just about impossible.

A: The good news is that you don't have to exercise for 60 consecutive minutes. Current research shows that even moderate exercise broken into segments can have a significant effect on health and fitness. Break up your activity time into smaller segments of 15 or 30 minutes each. For example, if walking is the activity, you could walk for 15 minutes before work, 30 minutes at lunchtime, and another 15 minutes after dinner. This approach also reduces or eliminates the need to devote time to travel and changing clothes.

And if even these modifications don't work, you can still park your car farther from the office and walk to the building, climb the stairs twice during the day, walk to another department instead of calling or writing an e-mail, or walk to lunch. You might even consider holding a walking meeting with a colleague during which you discuss business.

Another option for managing frequency and duration is to increase the intensity of your workout to a vigorous level but cut the duration in half (to 75 minutes per week). Obviously, you save time with this plan, but it works only if you maintain the higher intensity throughout.

A third alternative is to use an equivalent mix of moderate and vigorous aerobic activity. In this regard, one particularly effective and efficient form of aerobic activity is called *interval training*. This approach simply divides your aerobic activity into intervals of hard and easy exertion. For example, imagine running fast for 3 minutes, then walking briskly for 3 minutes, and then repeating the sequence a few more times. The result is a vigorous but manageable and perhaps fun aerobic activity that stimulates more fitness improvement in less time. Most sports, games, and fun physical activities (e.g., soccer, basketball, tennis) involve intervals of high-intensity activity followed by lower-intensity activity. You might try incorporating interval training as a variation, or you might enjoy using it on a regular basis.

The choice between these three options is, of course, up to you, and your decision should be dictated by your current fitness level, the types of activities you prefer, and the available time. Any of these three plans will produce a significant effect on your personal energy level, and none is clearly better than the others.

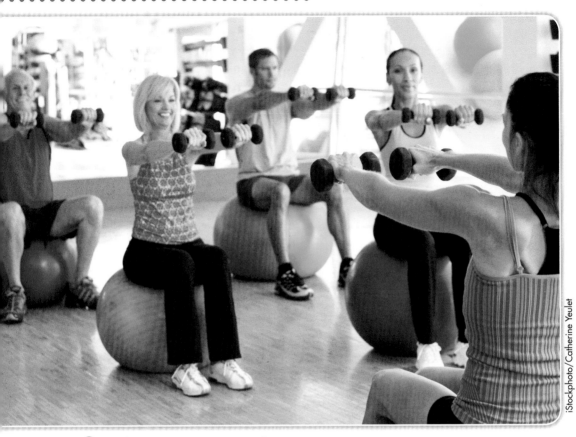

Strength training in a group can boost your motivation.

Don't forget your recovery days. On these days, you should warm up, stretch, or do some lower-intensity activities.

• Strength training should be done twice a week on nonconsecutive days in order to produce improvement but also allow for recovery. Don't strength-train daily unless you have been advised by a physical therapist or physician to do so in rehabilitating an injury. Strength training should work all the major muscle groups of your body, including legs, hips, chest, abdomen, shoulders, and arms. Chapter 9 provides more specific information, including descriptions and photographs, about doing strength training by adding resistance.

• Flexibility training can be done every day; in fact, if flexibility is a weakness for you, then you *should* do light warm-up and stretching activity on a daily basis. At a minimum, you should stretch after you have finished your physical activity. The American College of Sports Medicine recommends flexibility training at least 2 or 3 days per week, including either static or dynamic techniques, depending on your other movement activities. Refer to chapter 9 for specific recommendations and instructions for flexibility training.

Intensity

Next, let's consider the aerobic intensity of your chosen sport or physical activity. The intensity of aerobic activity can be judged in three ways; if possible, use all three methods to regularly assess the intensity of your activity. While the heart rate monitor is the most accurate of the three methods, if one isn't available, the other two more subjective methods are more convenient. The Borg scale is also useful if heart rate measurement is difficult or you are on medication that alters normal heart rate response to physical stress.

- *Use your heart rate.* To estimate your recommended maximum heart rate, subtract your age from 220; for example, if you are 45 years old, subtract 45 from 220 to arrive at an estimated maximum heart rate of 175. Then perform two calculations. First, figure out the range of heart rates that represents 60 to 70 percent of your estimated maximum heart rate; this range indicates your target heart rate zone for *moderate* activity. For example, the 60 percent to 70 percent range for an estimated maximum heart rate of 175 would be 105 (175 $\times$ 0.6) to 123 (175 $\times$ 0.7). Second, figure the range that represents 80 percent to 90 percent of your estimated maximum heart rate; this range indicates your target heart rate zone for *vigorous* activity. For an estimated maximum heart rate of 175, this range would be 140 (175 $\times$ 0.8) to 158 (175 $\times$ 0.9). Thus your target heart rate zone for moderate activity would be 105 to 123, and your target zone for vigorous activity would be 140 to 158.

We strongly recommend that you use a personal heart rate monitor to accurately and easily monitor your rate during activity. (Alternatively, you can measure your pulse for 10 seconds and multiply the result by 6.)

Frequently Asked Questions

Q: I play tennis three times a week, but the intensity seems to be quite low. Should I switch to another sport, or is it just me?

A: Many sports can be played at various levels of intensity. If you enjoy a sport but want a better workout, analyze what is not working. In tennis, if two evenly matched players can keep the ball in play for a number of successive hits during a rally or point, then both players will probably work fairly hard. But if each rally or point involves only one or two shots, then the activity involves little movement challenge; instead, you mostly just retrieve balls from nearby courts or from the back fence. If your tennis is not active enough, you'd probably benefit from some coaching to improve your hitting consistency and control of the ball. At the intermediate and advanced levels of play, most players get a very intense workout from 60 or 90 minutes of singles or doubles play.

- *Use the talk test.* Your ability to hold a conversation during even vigorous aerobic activity serves as a reasonable indicator that the intensity is not too high. If you cannot hold a conversation, reduce the intensity.

- *Use the Borg scale.* Most people find this tool easy to use, and research has shown it to be a fairly accurate measure of intensity. The exertion scale allows to you to rate your feelings of exertion on a scale of 6 to 20, with 6 representing rest and 20 representing exhaustion. A rating of 7 to 12 indicates intensity ranging from very light to fairly light. A rating of 13 or 14 indicates somewhat heavy intensity, and ratings of 15 and 16 indicate a hard workout. You can consider 13 and 14 as representing moderate activity and 15 and 16 as representing vigorous activity (American College of Sports Medicine, 2009). A rating of 17 indicates very heavy intensity and is too much; at this point you will be unable to pass the talk test, and you should reduce the intensity. Strive to exercise somewhere in the range of 13 to 16—that is, somewhat hard to hard—in order to reap the greatest benefit from your physical activity.

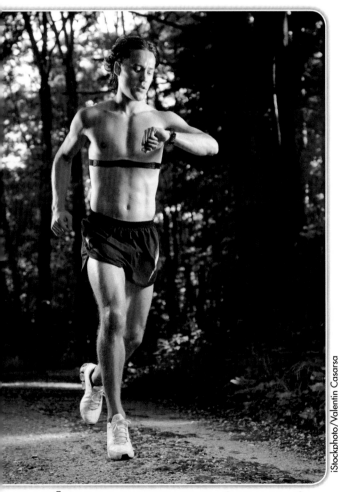

Now, let's consider the intensity of your strength and flexibility training. For strength training, choose a weight or resistance that you can lift with correct form and technique (i.e., slowly, under control, through the full range of motion, and with an out-breath upon exertion) for 8 to 12 repetitions. If you can perform 15 repetitions, it may be time to increase the weight or resistance. Perform 1 or 2 sets of 8 to 10 exercises, making sure to work each muscle group (chest, back, legs, shoulders, arms, abdominals, and lower back).

For flexibility training, stretch slowly and under control to the point of mild discomfort or even just a feeling of tightness in the muscles or tendons. Never stretch to the point of pain. Remember to breathe normally and hold each stretch for 15 to 30 seconds. Perform 2 to 4 repetitions of each stretch and at least one stretch for each muscle group.

iStockphoto/Valentin Casarsa

A heart rate monitor measures the intensity of your activity.

SAMPLE PLAN ANALYSIS

Now it's time to test your analytical skills by examining several typical plans for physical activity. Read the personal prescriptions that Maria, James, and Lisa have developed, then use the information presented in this chapter to compare their plans with the recommended standards and judge whether each plan is likely to help the person achieve his or her aims.

Maria's Plan

Maria has chosen the following sports and activities: coed volleyball once a week, tennis once a week, and walking 3 days a week followed by flexibility training. She will do each of these activities with two of her best friends, and the coed volleyball includes the spouses of all three women. What is she missing?

You may have noticed that Maria has included no activity to address muscular strength and endurance in her plan. Depending on her intensity of effort, she may be meeting the other three components of fitness just fine, but she is missing one vitally important area.

James' Plan

James has chosen the following sports and activities: golf once a week, swimming three times a week in his backyard pool, and weightlifting in his garage on Saturdays and Sundays. He plays golf with whoever else shows up on Saturday mornings, and the other activities are done alone. What is your evaluation of James' plan?

Our concerns focus first on James' plan to do 2 consecutive days of weight work; in addition, because he uses the term *weightlifting* we believe that he may plan to lift heavy weights and concentrate primarily on building strength or even on bodybuilding. We prefer the term *strength training*, which means overloading various muscles to improve both strength and endurance. At the very least, James needs to allow for at least 1 day of recovery between the two sessions.

Second, swimming is an excellent aerobic exercise, but since it is not weight bearing (your buoyancy in the water reduces the work you have to do) it does not serve the same purpose as walking, jogging, or other similar activities. We need to do weight-bearing activity in order to develop and maintain strong bones.

Third, upon talking with James, we found out that he rides a golf cart for his weekly game on the links, thus limiting the amount of exercise he gets while playing. Finally, having met James, who is a gregarious guy, we believe that he would enjoy some pursuits that involve more social interaction during and after the activity. Indeed, he may come to dread his individual workout after a few weeks.

(continued)

Sample Plan Analysis   *(continued)*

Lisa's Plan

Lisa has gained about 25 pounds (11 kg) since delivering her last child and simply needs to get to the gym. She plans to hire a personal trainer to plan a program for her that addresses all four components of fitness. Because she has returned to work and now has a newborn to care for, her time is more limited than ever. She hopes to go to the gym twice a week at 5:30 a.m. when her husband can be home with their children.

Her biggest problem is that she has never worked out at a gym before and has felt very anxious about her appearance since adding the extra weight. Most of the customers are male, and Lisa is a bit shy about exercising around men. What are some alternatives that might ease her anxiety?

Our take on this plan is that it is very ambitious. Lisa's life is extremely busy, and we'd rate her chances of getting to the gym twice a week as moderate at best. Even then, the frequency is insufficient for her to succeed in her weight loss plan. In view of Lisa's self-consciousness, a better option might be to join a group exercise session with other women in similar situations. This approach would reduce the pressure while allowing Lisa to socialize outside the home. A second recommendation is for her to consider some follow-up activity sessions at home where she and her spouse can divide the time. Using exercise tapes, an exercise ball, resistance bands, or simple walks around the block might be a better fit for her schedule and responsibilities. Finally, we'd recommend that Lisa get some nutritional counseling or even join a group to help her modify her diet. If weight loss is the goal, exercise alone is not enough.

Your Plan

Once you have critiqued the plans developed by Maria, James, and Lisa, use the same criteria to carefully evaluate your own plan. Are you happy with your choices? Will they get you where you want to go? Do you need advice from a professional to help you modify your plan?

FINALIZING YOUR PLAN FOR SPORT AND PHYSICAL ACTIVITY

Congratulations! You have developed a sport and activity plan for the next 2 weeks. Now, to the best of your ability, fill out figure 8.1 in order to develop a physical activity schedule for yourself. Note each physical activity, the day(s) and time(s) you will do it, and the duration; in addition, indicate whether the intensity will be high, moderate, or low. As you begin, you may have to adjust some days due to health issues or work or family demands, but make a good faith effort to complete your 2-week plan as shown on your chart. After that, you can modify the frequency, duration, or intensity as needed. Remember to include *rest days* on your calendar, and make sure that your duration and intensity of activity remain in line with recommendations (presented earlier in the chapter) by the Centers for Disease Control and Prevention and the American College of Sports Medicine.

Once you begin to execute your plan, it is critical that you keep a simple daily log of results to hold yourself accountable and track the results of your activity. This record will be the key document you use to evaluate your program after 2 weeks and plan how to continue moving forward. Don't rely on your memory after a busy 2 weeks to recall what you accomplished on each day. Write down the results each day as you complete your workout.

Consider sharing your daily log with a trusted friend, a professional coach, your spouse, or even your kids. If you choose to share your results with someone you do not see regularly, you can use e-mail to do so every few days, weekly, or at the end of each 2-week period. Exposing our performance to another person can be a powerful motivator for many of us; it can also serve as a terrific measure of accountability.

FIGURE 8.1	**Sport and Physical Activity Schedule**				
DATES:					
Day	**Activity**	**Duration**	**Intensity**	**Score**	**Fun**
WEEK 1					
Sunday					
Monday					
Tuesday					
Wednesday					
Thursday					
Friday					
Saturday					
WEEK 2					
Sunday					
Monday					
Tuesday					
Wednesday					
Thursday					
Friday					
Saturday					

From R. Woods and C. Jordan with the Human Performance Institute, 2010, *Energy every day* (Champaign, IL: Human Kinetics).

As you progress through your schedule, give yourself a daily score from 0 to 5 (5 for highest) to indicate whether you achieved your goals for that day. If you completed the activity as planned, your score should be a 5. If you did no activity, assign a score of 0 for that day.

The last column in the figure is critical. Make a check mark here if you had *fun*. Remember, your definition of fun is unique to you. If you did not have fun, consider why that may be. Do you need to change your activity, or perhaps change your attitude toward it? Perhaps your definition of fun was inappropriate or too narrow for you?

FINAL INSTRUCTIONS AND ADVICE

Now you have a plan for getting started. Before beginning, study the information in chapter 9 to increase your understanding of how to properly warm up and cool down, how to use resistance training to build muscular strength and endurance, and how to use both dynamic and static stretching to improve your flexibility. Planning a course of action is an important first step because you now have a clear path to follow. You can begin on any day of the week, but we suggest beginning on a weekend day since you are likely to have more free time then and thus can't blame work for interfering!

Here are some final words of advice for you to hold in mind on the first day and throughout these first 2 weeks.

• *Start slowly and ease into the routine.* This is particularly important if you have been inactive for some time; nothing is more discouraging than to end up stiff, sore, or even injured after just a day or two.

• *"No pain, no gain" is a poor philosophy.* Make every effort to enjoy the activities you've chosen, and perform them at a comfortable level, especially in the beginning.

• *Consult a professional if you are uncertain about your plan.* Be sure that your planned activities fall within your ability range, that you use sound technique, and that the activities pose little risk of injury. If you need coaching on technique, join a group or engage a professional coach for private assessment and recommendations. Poor technique in strength training, for example, may exacerbate a weakness or lead to injury. Be sure to study the next chapter for more specific guidance on strength and flexibility training before you begin.

• *Secure good equipment before you begin.* That old tennis racket, set of golf clubs, or pair of running shoes may have been state-of-the-art 10 years ago, but today's sports equipment is light years beyond. Do yourself a favor by borrowing or buying good equipment from the start. It'll make you feel better and more eager, and the activity will be more fun.

• *Keep a record of your workouts* as a motivational technique. At the end of each day or week, look back at what you've accomplished. If you need someone to help you be accountable, show that person your plan and your results on a regular basis. Choose a trusted friend, spouse, or even your children. It's hard to admit to your 10-year-old that you've failed to perform!

• *Stick to your plan for the first 2 weeks,* then step back and assess. You may need to modify an activity, add something, improve your warm-up or cool-down routine, or engage a professional coach for guidance.

• *Increase the intensity of activity* as you develop greater confidence and skill.

• *Test yourself again after 6 weeks of activity.* It is unlikely that you will see significant changes before then. Use the same tests and conduct them exactly as you did in your initial testing. Evaluate your results and adjust your activity routine accordingly.

TIPS for High Energy

• The goal of this chapter is to help you develop a 2-week schedule of sports and physical activity.

• Gather all of your previously developed information to use in planning your activity choices.

• Consider your sport and activity plan in light of your fitness test results from chapter 5.

• Determine the frequency, duration, and intensity you need in order to achieve your personal goals for activity.

• Complete figure 8.1, your personal sport and physical activity schedule for the next 2 weeks.

• Review the final instructions and get ready to begin! Your final step before beginning is to read chapter 9 (Putting Your Plan into Action).

PART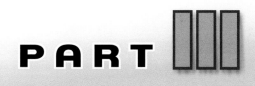

YOUR ACTION PLAN

PUTTING YOUR PLAN INTO ACTION

You're almost ready to begin your personal program of sport and physical activity. Before you start exercising, however, you need a few more tools to make your physical activity productive and enjoyable.

In this chapter, we share with you the benefits of learning to breathe properly, both for relaxation and to maximize your workout. We also offer recommendations for warm-up and dynamic stretching before your workout activity and for cool-down and stretching after the activity. These routines prepare, prime and protect the body and thus enhance your enjoyment, help you avoid injury, and ensure that your activity time is both efficient and productive.

The chapter also introduces you to the essential methods of using resistance in strength training. In simple terms, we show multiple options for accomplishing the same goal of building muscular strength and endurance. We urge you to try several methods in order to add variety to your training and to avail yourself of the special benefits provided by each method. You may be limited by time, space, or cost, but at least one of the suggested methods will work for you in any situation.

Finally, we help you prepare mentally and emotionally to embark on a new journey toward a higher level of physical fitness. Using years of accumulated wisdom from working with people just like you, we offer recommendations about how you might think and feel as you begin your program. Adjusting your attitude may be the key to success.

HEAVY BREATHING

Breathing is a natural, automatic, and vital body function that transports oxygen throughout your body and removes carbon dioxide. Your rate and depth of breathing are normally adjusted without conscious thought. After all, you've been breathing unconsciously ever since birth, so why change now?

The fact is that people who speak to a group, sing, play a wind instrument, perform in front of an audience, or participate in sport or physical activity soon realize the need to voluntarily control their breathing and regulate it to fit the needs of the moment. You can change both the rate and depth of your breathing in order to relax, lower your heart rate, reduce muscle tension, lower your blood pressure, and respond more effectively to stress. Indeed, proper breathing allows you to fill every muscle, tendon, and tissue with the oxygen it needs in order to function, grow, or heal.

When we feel stressed or in danger, our breathing becomes shallower, shorter, more rapid, and irregular. At times of high stress or emergency, our sympathetic nervous system triggers the "fight-or-flight" response, which increases our heart rate, blood pressure, muscle tension, and respiratory rate. Though helpful in an emergency, this response is undesirable on a daily basis because it just adds to our tension and stress. Instead, we need to voluntarily control our breathing; specifically, we need to engage in deep breathing that allows us to recover our personal energy and function more effectively.

Optimal breathing begins from the diaphragm, not the chest, and deep breathing exercises using only the abdomen (i.e., belly breathing) help you develop better breathing habits, both at rest and during physical activity. To practice deep breathing, place one hand on your abdomen just above your navel and inhale smoothly and slowly through your nose. Concentrate on filling the lower portion of your lungs and pushing your abdomen out, without raising your chest or shoulders. When you feel that your lungs are completely full, hold the breath for 2 seconds, then slowly release it through your mouth until your lungs feel completely empty. Aim to exhale twice as long as you inhale and keep your breaths at a steady rate. Draw your abdomen in to force out every last bit of air and wait 2 seconds before you begin another deep, slow breath. Continue this pattern for at least 1 minute.

As you exhale, consciously allow all of your muscles to relax and focus on your breathing pattern. It may be helpful to close your eyes in order to remove distractions. You should practice these breathing techniques while sitting upright, but you can also do them while lying on your back (supine position), and while lying on your front (prone position). The supine and prone positions will particularly help you see and feel your abdomen move in and out.

At the end of a minute, chances are that your blood pressure will be lower, you head clearer, and your muscles more relaxed. If you have not reached this state, try using the same patterns for another minute or two.

When you are performing a physical activity, your breathing patterns are crucial to the movement and to replenishing your supply of oxygen and removing carbon dioxide. If you engage in slow, rhythmic breathing (leading with the abdomen) during continuous activity (e.g., riding a bicycle, walking, or running), you will be better able to remain relaxed and energetic.

If you are performing sudden power movements (e.g., swinging a golf club or tennis racket or lifting a weight), be sure to *exhale* during the movement and *inhale* during the recovery phase. You may often notice that athletes violently expel air when performing a vigorous move, and this expulsion may sound more

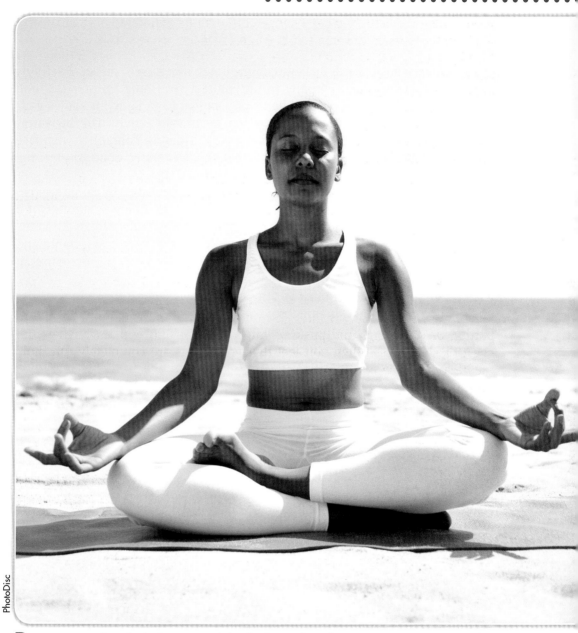

PhotoDisc

Practice controlling both the rate and depth of your breathing.

like a grunt or cry of pain than an exhalation. Understand, however, that this is a natural, healthy move as they exert sudden force and effort. Inexperienced athletes who reverse the process by *inhaling* when performing a strenuous move simply cause their muscles to become tense and unnecessarily increase overall effort.

WARM-UP AND DYNAMIC STRETCHING

You absolutely *must* warm up before engaging in any type of physical activity. Think about it this way: Prepare, prime, protect. Warming up prepares and primes your body for activity and helps protect you from injury. It allows your body to perform at an optimal level once you begin your activity. During warm-up, you want to raise your body temperature by 1 degree Fahrenheit, increase blood flow, and increase your metabolic activity. Generally, once you feel the first drop of perspiration, you are probably warmed up.

We recommend performing a general warm-up, followed by dynamic stretching. As a guide, we recommend that you warm up by doing 5 minutes of a simple, aerobic activity (e.g., walking, jogging, doing gentle strokes in water, riding a stationary bike). The activity should be aerobic yet comfortable and of low intensity. Try to involve your entire body—for example, by using an elliptical or rowing machine or by swimming.

Once you have raised your body temperature, we suggest that you consider doing some additional dynamic movements typical of the activity you have chosen to perform. Simply put, we suggest that you mimic the movements you are about to perform but do them in a controlled and comfortable manner. For example, if you will be playing a sport that involves quick bursts of running, then you should do dynamic stretches that prime your feet, ankles, and knees as well as the supporting muscles of your calves, quadriceps, and hamstrings. Following are a few options (perform each for a minimum of 20 seconds).

HEEL-TO-TOE WALK

Walk while exaggerating the heel-to-toe motion by striking the ground with your heel first; your toes should be held high off the ground. Next, roll onto the ball of your foot, then onto your toes. Finally, lift your heel high off the ground as you push forward for the next step.

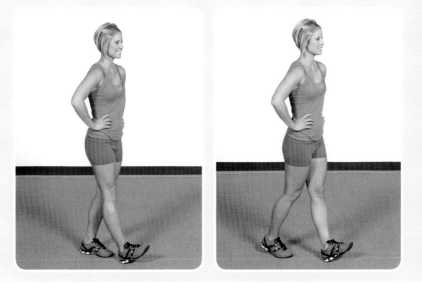

WALKING HIGH-KNEES

Walk while raising each knee toward your chest and as high off the ground as possible as you take each step forward. You can progress from here to running high knees, if appropriate for you and your intended activity.

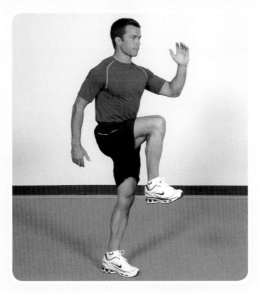

SIDEWAYS WALK

Walk sideways by first standing with your feet together and stepping to the left with your left foot. Then step in the same direction with your right foot to bring your feet together again. Continue. Repeat this exercise while leading with your right foot.

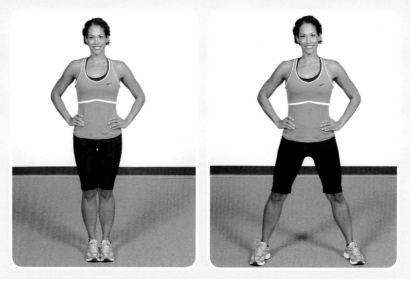

WALKING LUNGE

Stand with your feet shoulder-width apart and your knees slightly bent. Holding an upright posture, take a big step forward and bend both knees to lower your body toward the ground. Make sure that your back stays straight, your knees do not pass beyond your toes, and you are looking straight forward. Raise your body and bring your back foot forward to the front foot and repeat while leading with the opposite foot. You can progress from here to a sideways walking lunge, if appropriate for you and your intended activity.

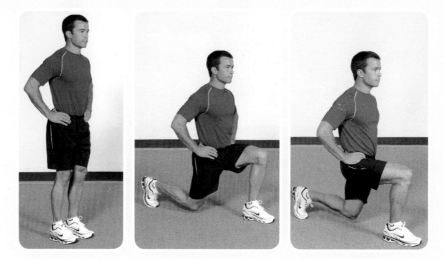

WALKING STRAIGHT-LEG KICKS

Walk while kicking each leg up in front of you. Aim to keep your leg straight and touch your toes with the hand of the opposite side arm.

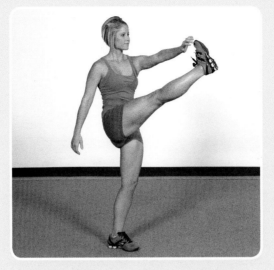

RUNNING BUTT-KICKS

Run slowly and aim to flick or kick your heels as a high as you can behind you (toward your glutes).

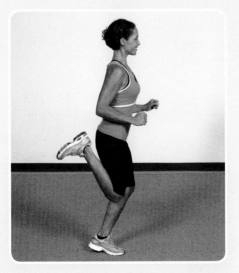

Sports that involve striking skills (e.g., golf, softball, tennis, racquetball, squash, badminton, and volleyball) require that your upper body be prepared for the aggressive twisting and turning that you will do in order to strike an object. Perform each of the following dynamic stretches for at least 30 seconds.

WRIST FLEXION AND EXTENSION

Stand with your feet shoulder-width apart, your knees slightly bent, and your arms relaxed by your sides (with the palms of your hands facing forward). Curl (flex) your hands toward your forearms, then straighten (extend) your hands back out. Repeat the flexion and extension. You can also add wrist circles, clockwise and counterclockwise.

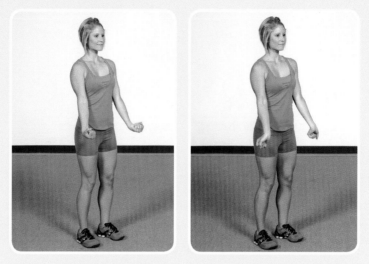

ARM CIRCLES

Standing with your feet shoulder-width apart, your knees slightly bent, and your arms relaxed by your sides, raise your straight arms forward and above your head. Then, lower your arms out to the side and back to the starting position to complete the arm circle. Rotate your arms in both directions (forward and backward).

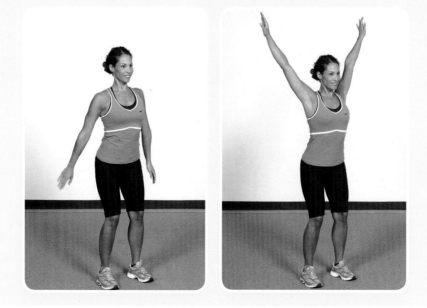

STANDING TRUNK ROTATIONS

Stand with your feet shoulder-width apart, your knees slightly bent, and your arms relaxed by your sides. Gently twist your torso and swing your arms in one direction, then in the other direction.

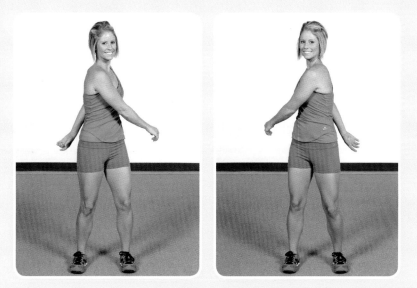

HIP CIRCLES

Stand with your feet shoulder-width apart, your knees slightly bent, and your hands on your hips. Make a circle by moving your hips in one direction. Once finished, rotate your hips in the other direction.

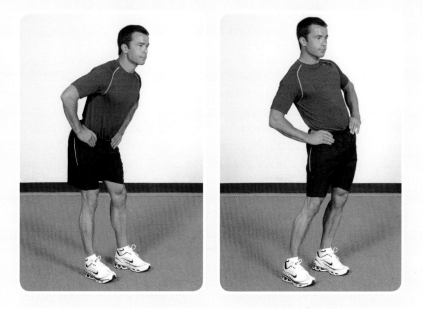

Warming up for strength training should include some of the same exercises you'll use during your workout per se but with much less resistance during the warm-up. You might even complete a circuit of strength activities using light weights and only a few repetitions before you begin your workout. A quick way to specifically warm up for a resistance training workout is to perform one set of the chest press, back row, and leg press exercises using a light weight. These three exercises incorporate all the major muscle groups and joints. Alternatively, just perform one set of each exercise you choose using a light weight before your challenging set.

Warm-up for most skill sports should also include several trials of performing each skill to be used during the game. Baseball players should hit, field, throw, and run. Tennis players should hit all the shots they plan to use in the match. Basketball players should dribble, pass, shoot, and defend. Volleyball players should serve, pass, dig, and spike.

The time you take for warm-up is crucial, but it need not consume many minutes. Usually, a complete routine can be accomplished by doing 10 minutes of efficient movements—for example, 5 minutes of general warm-up followed by 5 minutes of dynamic stretches or resistance movements with light weights (depending on the activity you will engage in). As you age, it might be wise to make your warm-up and dynamic stretching period a bit longer. We generally become less fit as we age, largely as a result of diminishing activity, and our muscles, tendons, and ligaments become worn and brittle; consequently, it is wise to spend more time preparing gradually for moderately vigorous exertion by warming up.

COOL-DOWN AND FLEXIBILITY TRAINING

Equally important as the warm-up is the cool-down after physical activity. In many sports, it is almost a tradition that at the end of the contest the participants head for refreshments (usually drinks and snacks). They overlook the importance of allowing the body to cool down naturally, and they miss the opportunity of stretching for flexibility. Don't make this mistake. Instead, make sure that every workout includes a cool-down period and time for stretching.

The cool-down period allows blood to be redistributed gradually and evenly around the body, thus preventing blood from pooling in the muscles (which can cause light-headedness and dizziness, among other things). The most effective way to cool down at the end of your activity is probably to continue exercising but at a much lower intensity. This approach helps your muscles recover by flushing waste products, metabolizing and removing excess lactic acid, and replenishing precious glucose. We recommend that you cool down for at least 5 minutes, then, ideally, do a stretching session while your muscles and tendons are warm and more pliable. Stretching helps you maintain and improve flexibility (and being flexible can help prevent injury); it also releases muscle tension and has a temporary analgesic effect that makes you feel good afterward (if not during!).

When performing a static stretch, hold the stretch at the point of tightness (or, at most, mild discomfort—but not pain) for 15 to 30 seconds. Be sure to inhale and exhale slowly to help you relax the muscles as you stretch; breathe normally as you hold the stretch. It is recommended that you do equal stretching on both sides of your body. Ideally, perform 2 to 4 repetitions of each of the following stretches; if you are short on time, 1 repetition will still be beneficial. It is important to remember not to bounce during a stretch—simply hold the position for the recommended time.

If you perform stretching exercises after aerobic or strength training sessions, that may be sufficient to enhance your general flexibility. One advantage of stretching after these sessions is that your muscles, tendons, and joints are fully warm and ready to stretch. If you need additional stretching even on rest days to keep yourself limber, relaxed, and in good posture, then by all means add some flexibility training on any day. Just remember to warm up your body before doing stretching of any kind.

MODIFIED HURDLER STRETCH

➤ *Muscles Worked* Hamstrings

➤ *Execution* Sitting on the floor, extend your left leg in front of you and bend your right leg, placing your right foot against your left knee. Keeping your back straight, bend at the hips, lean forward, and reach with your left hand toward your left foot, exhaling as you do so. Stop at the point of tightness or mild discomfort and hold for 15 to 30 seconds. Breathe normally as you hold the stretch. Release slowly and return to the starting position. Repeat for the right side.

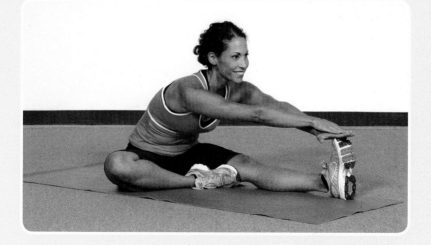

BUTTERFLY

≫ *Muscles Worked*   Groin

≫ *Execution*   Sitting on the floor with your knees bent and your feet flat on the floor, allow your knees to drop to either side of your body. Keep your back straight and hold your feet with your hands. Gently push your knees farther to either side with your elbows. Stop at the point of tightness or mild discomfort and hold for 15 to 30 seconds. Breathe normally as you hold the stretch. Release slowly and return to the starting position.

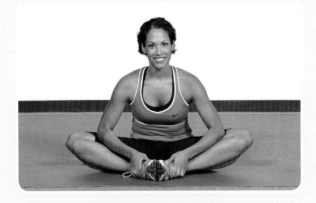

CAT STRETCH

≫ *Muscles Worked*   Low back

≫ *Execution*   Position yourself on your hands and knees, with your hands directly below your shoulders and your knees directly below your hips. Gently tuck your chin to your chest, draw your abdominals in toward the spine, and arch your back like an angry cat. Stop at the point of tightness or mild discomfort and hold for 15 to 30 seconds. Breathe normally as you hold the stretch. Release slowly and return to the starting position.

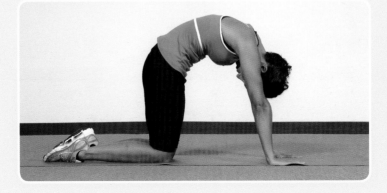

CHILD'S POSE

≫ *Muscles Worked*   Back

≫ *Execution*   Assume a kneeling position on the floor, then sit back on your calves. Lower your torso toward the floor and reach as far forward as you can along the floor with extended arms, while staying in the seated position. Stop at the point of tightness or mild discomfort and hold for 15 to 30 seconds. Breathe normally as you hold the stretch. Release slowly and return to the starting position.

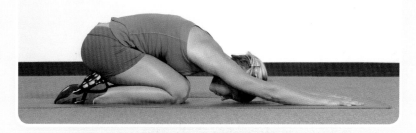

CALF STRETCH

≫ *Muscles Worked*   Calves

≫ *Execution*   Position yourself on your hands and knees, with your hands directly below your shoulders and your knees directly below your hips. Extend your left leg behind you, plant your toes against the floor, and, keeping your leg straight, push back with your hands to move your left heel back. Stop at the point of tightness or mild discomfort and hold for 15 to 30 seconds. Breathe normally as you hold the stretch. Release slowly and return to the starting position.

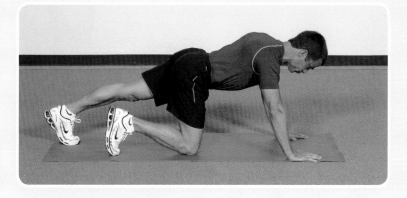

STANDING QUAD STRETCH

≫ *Muscles Worked*   Quadriceps

≫ *Execution*   Standing with your feet shoulder-width apart, your knees slightly bent, and your arms relaxed by your sides, bring your right foot behind your glutes with your right hand, keeping your knees together and your body upright. Stop at the point of tightness or mild discomfort and hold for 15 to 30 seconds. Breathe normally as you hold the stretch. Release slowly and return to the starting position. Repeat for the left side.

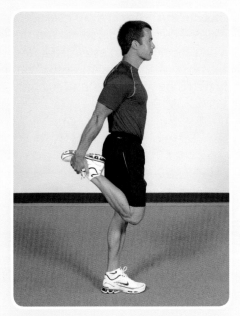

REACH-ABOVE

≫ *Muscles Worked*   Back and biceps

≫ *Execution*   Standing with your feet shoulder-width apart and your knees slightly bent, interlock your hands (with palms facing out) and extend your arms above your head. Stop at the point of tightness or mild discomfort and hold for 15 to 30 seconds. Breathe normally as you hold the stretch. Release slowly and return to the starting position.

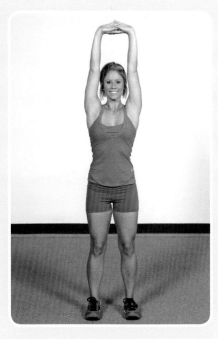

REACH-BEHIND

≫ *Muscles Worked*   Chest and shoulders

≫ *Execution*   Standing with your feet shoulder-width apart and your knees slightly bent, interlock your hands (with palms facing in) and extend your arms behind you, keeping your body in an upright posture. Stop at the point of tightness or mild discomfort and hold for 15 to 30 seconds. Breathe normally as you hold the stretch. Release slowly and return to the starting position.

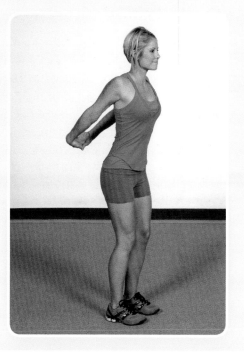

REACH-IN-FRONT

≫ *Muscles Worked*   Back and shoulders

≫ *Execution*   Standing with your feet shoulder-width apart and your knees slightly bent, interlock your hands (with palms facing out) and extend your arms in front out of you, allowing your upper back to round. Stop at the point of tightness or mild discomfort and hold for 15 to 30 seconds. Breathe normally as you hold the stretch. Release slowly and return to the starting position.

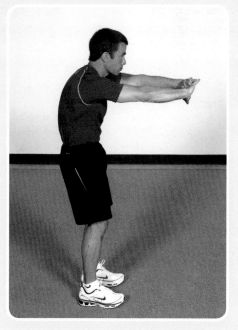

OVERHEAD TRICEPS

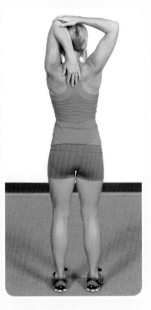

> *Muscles Worked*   Triceps and shoulders

> *Execution*   Standing with your feet shoulder-width apart and your knees slightly bent, extend your left arm above your head and bend it to lower your left hand behind your head and between your shoulder blades. Using your right hand, gently pull on your upper left arm. Stop at the point of tightness or mild discomfort and hold for 15 to 30 seconds. Breathe normally as you hold the stretch. Release slowly and return to the starting position. Repeat for the right side.

MUSCULAR STRENGTH AND ENDURANCE TRAINING

Strength training is vital to your overall fitness routine. Here are some facts about what happens to our muscular strength and endurance as we age, unless we continue to train our muscles.

- After age 25, you lose 4 percent of your muscle mass every 10 years until you reach age 40.
- After age 40, you lose 1 percent every year, for a total of *10 percent* in 10 years. This means that the average person loses 16 percent of muscle mass by age 50 and 26 percent by age 60.
- The greatest loss of muscular strength occurs in the lower body—in the lower back, buttocks, thighs, and calves.
- Unless you continue to train your muscles, you will also lose endurance, flexibility, and ability to process oxygen effectively. In addition, your chances of injury increase exponentially.

We have two primary types of muscle fibers, and they are usually referred to as *fast-twitch* and *slow-twitch* fibers. Fast-twitch fibers contract quickly and forcefully. They provide power and strength and help us engage in explosive activities that demand jumping, moving fast, and lifting heavy weights. These fibers tire more quickly than do slow-twitch fibers, which contract more slowly and provide muscular endurance. Slow-twitch fibers allow us to be active for long periods of time. Fortunately, the effect of aging on slow-twitch fibers is less dramatic than on fast-twitch fibers.

As we age, we see a 25 to 50 percent reduction in the number and size of fast-twitch fibers, especially in the back, quadriceps, hamstrings, and calves. This decline begins after age 25 and continues at a similar rate to that of muscle mass loss. Thus, if you want to maintain at least some explosiveness of movement, you simply must continue to train those muscles.

The good news for you is that through muscular strength and endurance training, you can reverse some effects of aging and significantly reduce your loss of strength and endurance. Perhaps even better, strength training also improves your bone health, posture, and flexibility and increases your metabolism, thus helping reduce body fat.

In the rest of this chapter, we explain, in simple terms, the basic principles of resistance training and how to perform a resistance training workout that is safe, effective, and efficient. We then present a variety of resistance training exercises organized into workouts, complete with instructions for performing the exercises, listing of the muscle(s) affected by each exercise, and a photo illustration of the exercise.

Frequently Asked Questions

Q: I'm female and am not really into developing prominent muscles. Should I be doing strength training?

A: Yes, absolutely. Generally, females are not genetically predisposed to developing large muscles and they have less of the male hormone (testosterone) that allows males to do so. In fact, some males will not develop bulging muscles no matter how much they work out. It is worth noting that a muscle gets stronger before it gets bigger and that some resistance training is needed just to maintain your current muscular size and strength!

The point is to include muscular strength and endurance training in your activity regimen—no matter your age, sex, or history of physical activity. It is simply one of the four elements of fitness that cannot be ignored.

Resistance Training Principles

Resistance training simply involves applying a load or resistance to your muscles that they are unaccustomed to handling. The resulting stress on the muscles stimulates them to repair and grow stronger (and possibly bigger, too) when you recover after your workout. The key is to apply just the right amount of stress—too much stress causes injury, and too little produces no improvement. Here's a simple way to remember this principle: Pain is too much stress, comfort is too little, and discomfort is just right.

The good news here is that if you challenge your muscles, you also challenge your joints and bones. Consequently, resistance training is an excellent way to maintain a healthy, strong body that makes everyday activities easier to do and is more resilient against injury. You will be less likely to sustain an injury and in the case that you do, the healing process will be accelerated. Another benefit of resistance training is that even several hours after your workout, your metabolism will be at a high level and burning calories; you simply don't get that benefit from aerobic activities.

Resistance training may be more accessible than you first realize. Almost any pushing, pulling, carrying, or lifting of a challenging load or resistance offers potential as a resistance workout. Lifting dumbbells in a gym and lifting children at home can have similar benefits! In the next section of this chapter, we present a variety of resistance training options, or types, and detail their pros and cons. We suggest that you try multiple methods in order to vary your routine and to ensure that when you travel you can use any training option that is available.

Intensity, Duration, and Frequency

A safe, effective, and efficient resistance training workout meets specific criteria in terms of frequency, duration, and intensity. You may recall these terms from chapter 8, and we'd like to revisit them here.

Intensity refers to the amount of resistance or weight lifted; this amount must be sufficient to apply just the right degree of stress to your muscles. Remember, discomfort (not pain or comfort) is the goal. To ensure the right intensity, you should choose a weight that you can lift for 8 to 12 repetitions using the correct form and technique. The number of repetitions is simply the number of times you perform the exercise movement in succession without resting. Lifting a weight with correct form and technique means lifting slowly, under control, though the full range of motion, breathing normally as you do so, and breathing out during the exertion phase (the hardest part) of the exercise movement. As a guide, take about 3 seconds to lift the weight and about 3 seconds to lower the weight. If you forget to count, don't worry; just make sure you are controlling the weight at all times, rather than relying on momentum.

Muscular *strength* is crucial in many sports or activities. For example, sports such as softball and basketball require strength and power to swing a bat or jump for a ball. It would be wise to focus your resistance training on strength-building. To gear your resistance training for strength, choose a weight that you can lift for 8 to 10 repetitions.

Muscular *endurance* is most important in sports that rely upon your ability to perform repetitive movements without fatigue. Muscular endurance is essential for a long rally in tennis or repeated sprints in a soccer game. To emphasize muscular endurance, choose a weight that you can lift for 12 to 15 repetitions. Assess your muscular needs and tailor your resistance training accordingly. If you are not sure where to start, stick to the 8 to 12 repetition recommendation. It is a great place to start and will certainly provide you a good strength–muscular endurance balance.

If you cannot perform a minimum of 8 repetitions using the correct form and technique, consider the weight too heavy and decrease it slightly. (This is a somewhat conservative recommendation, but we would rather you be cautious than unrealistic about your current fitness status.) If you can perform more than 15 repetitions, consider the weight too light and increase it slightly. In general, we recommend that you perform 1 or 2 sets of each exercise in your workout. A set is one complete series of repetitions (e.g., 1 set of 12 repetitions).

The *duration* of your resistance training workout will vary, but as long as you exercise at the right intensity, workouts do not need to be prolonged in order to get results. In general, the more exercise you do, the greater benefit you receive (up to a point), but one big mistake made by many people is to reduce the intensity and work out for a longer time. This approach can lead to minimal or no fitness improvement since the most important factor—intensity—has been compromised! In general, we recommend that you allow 30 to 60 minutes for your workout; however, shorter workouts can still provide fitness improvements.

The *frequency* of your resistance training must allow your body to alternate intense workouts with rest and recovery. Aim to exercise each major muscle group twice a week. If you train all the major muscle groups during each workout, as we recommend, that means you will need to schedule just two days of working out during each week. You need to allow your muscles to recover after each workout, and this takes 48 hours or more, so make sure that your workouts are scheduled for nonconsecutive days. No more than 3 rest days are typically needed between workouts; for example, it is fine to schedule workouts on Monday and Thursday. If you are pressed for time on certain days and have, say, only 20 minutes available, you can train your upper body on one day and your lower body on the next, so long as you honor the principles regarding rest for each part of your body.

Key Muscle Groups to Train

The *major muscle groups* that should be trained twice a week are the chest, back, legs, shoulders, biceps, triceps, abdominals, and low back. Each workout should include at least one exercise for each of these muscle groups (or for each muscle group in either your upper or lower body, if you are splitting your workout into two sessions on different days). We include at least one exercise for each muscle group in each workout in the next section. If you omit any muscle groups from your workout, you will lose strength in the muscle itself (this is called *disuse atrophy*), regardless of how much cardiorespiratory exercise you do! (Cardiorespiratory activities are not intense enough to sufficiently challenge all the muscle fibers.)

Your *body core* is another muscle group you should train twice a week. The *core* simply means your torso. The muscles that make up the core include the abdominals and low back, as well as deeper muscles around the spine and pelvis. They must be strong, since they support and stabilize the spine while you sit, stand, walk, exercise, play sports, or lift weight. Training your core will increase overall stability, help prevent injury, and improve your sports performance.

To engage your core, try bracing your abdominal region as if you were a boxer taking a punch to the belly. At the least, we recommend that you engage your core in this way whenever you do resistance training. This serves as good practice and helps you improve core strength. In addition, we include exercises in the next section that specifically target core stability (see static body weight exercises such as plank, side plank, and bridge) and core strength (see stability ball exercises such as abdominal crunch and low-back extension).

Finally, the question arises: What type of resistance training should you do? Well, it depends on what is available to you and what you enjoy. In the next section, we provide a number of options for you to choose from.

Resistance Training Exercises

This section includes the specific exercises we recommend for building muscular strength and endurance. They are organized by type of equipment, and they range from the most common, accessible, convenient, and affordable to the more exotic, interesting, and, in many cases, safer machines. For each type, we present the pros and cons.

The six specific complete workouts that follow are identified by the method or equipment used:

- Body weight
- Resistance bands
- Stability balls
- Free weights (barbells and dumbbells)
- Cable machines
- Fixed-weight machines

Each workout is comprised of 12 exercises, works all the major muscle groups, and provides a complete workout. For each exercise, we list the muscle group involved, describe how to perform the exercise, and, where possible, offer a variation of the exercise.

Variety is a very important factor in long-term fitness improvement and prevention of boredom. We recommend that you try as many types of equipment as possible. Furthermore, you can mix and match the types of the equipment that you use in each workout. As long as you perform at least one exercise for each of the major muscle groups, you can pick a different selection of exercises every time.

Other options for strength and flexibility training include Pilates, yoga, tai chi, and other forms of martial arts. They all provide excellent variety in your routine and offer new skills that are fun and challenging. You do need to find a good teacher who is certified, experienced, and enthusiastic. Group workouts also give you an opportunity to meet new people, and the fact that you have made a commitment to a group may help motivate you to attend regularly. Of course, you can also perform the movements at home, either by yourself or while watching a video that demonstrates the moves.

Body Weight   Body-weight exercises can be performed just about anywhere, anytime. Although you are using only your own weight as the resistance, many of these body-weight exercises are surprisingly challenging. In addition, many of these exercises help you develop balance, skill, and coordination as they engage your core. As you become stronger, however, your body weight may not provide enough of a load for larger muscle groups such as the legs; in addition, if you rely on body weight, you are somewhat limited in the number of exercises you can do. Perform the body-weight exercises in this chapter in succession, with minimal or no rest between exercises, for a combined aerobic and resistance training circuit.

Resistance Bands   Resistance bands are easy to carry with you, and as with body weight exercises you can perform these exercises almost anywhere, anytime. Resistance bands are quite versatile, allowing many exercises and variations of exercises. As with body weight, many of these exercises help you develop balance, skill, and coordination while also engaging your core. Resistance bands are sold in different colors that indicate how flexible they are, and it is important to make sure you get the right resistance band for your strength level. For example, the Dyna Band brand produces four colors for different levels: the pink band offers light resistance and is recommended for injury rehabilitation; the green band is next and is recommended for beginners; the purple band offers more resistance than the green and is ideal for regular resistance trainers; and the gray band, which offers the most resistance, is recommended for athletes.

Stability Balls   The stability ball (or Swiss ball) is less portable than a resistance band, but it can be found in most fitness centers and is inexpensive to purchase for home use. Use of a stability ball engages your core muscles and, because you must maintain your balance on the ball throughout every exercise, it provides a great way to improve core stability and strength. The stability ball is also terrific for stretching exercises during flexibility training. Make sure you choose the ball size that is appropriate for your height. A good guideline to follow is that when you are seated on the ball, your hips and knees should be at right angles (90 degrees).

Free Weights (Dumbbells and Barbells)   Free weights (dumbbells and barbells) are found at most fitness centers and are often considered the best way to improve strength. This view is probably rooted in the fact that it takes a lot of effort to control and lift the weight—and more effort means greater gain. Once again, balance, skill, and coordination are required, and many of these exercises engage your core. However, you need a partner, and it would be expensive to set up all of this equipment at home. It can also be time consuming to load and unload weights for the various exercises.

Cable Machines   Cable machines are found at many, but not all, fitness centers. They are versatile and allow you to perform exercises in a variety of ways that mimic natural (functional) movements. These machines are particularly useful for engaging the core as you move. Cables pull the body out of balance and require the core to contract and re-stabilize the body, unlike typical weight machines that stabilize the body or free weights that are typically used on a stable platform like a bench. Cable machines are often used to help athletes improve their strength in ways tailored for their sport (e.g., for a golf swing, a swimming stroke, or a tennis backhand). Some cable machines can be quite expensive and may only be found at fitness centers; however, some cable equipment such as the Total Gym represents an affordable home-gym option.

Fixed-Weight Machines   Fixed-weight machines are great for beginners. You can use them to exercise safely on your own, and they require minimal balance, skill, and coordination. Workouts can be done very quickly, since you do not have to load and unload weights (as you do when using free weights). Fixed-weight machines can be found in almost every fitness center, but they are expensive and bulky and therefore not ideal for the home. In addition, since fixed-weight machines isolate muscle groups and thus reduce the need for balance and coordination, they fail to sufficiently address these important components of overall fitness.

JUMPING JACKS

➤ **Muscle Group Worked**
Legs

➤ **Execution** Start with your feet together. Begin the exercise by jumping so that both feet land out to the side while simultaneously raising your arms above your head. Then return to the starting position.

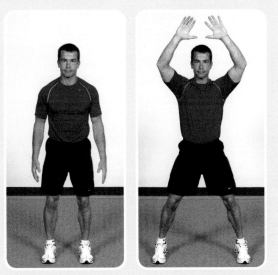

WALL SIT

➤ **Muscle Group Worked**   Legs

➤ **Execution**   Start by leaning against a wall with your shoulders and low back pressed against the wall. Lower your body into a sitting position while keeping your back against the wall. Make sure to keep your weight on your heels. Do not let your knees extend past your toes (your knees should be at a 90-degree angle). Hold this position for 30 seconds.

➤ **Variation**   For a more challenging intensity, perform the exercise by balancing on one leg (photo on right).

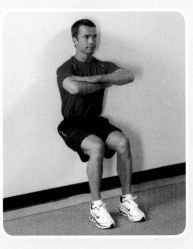 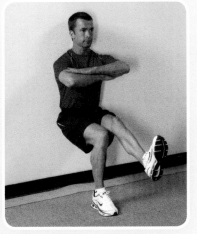

PUSH-UP

➤ *Muscle Group Worked*
Chest

➤ *Execution* Start by balancing on your hands and toes. Inhale and slowly lower yourself toward the floor by bending your arms at the elbows. Lower your body until your upper arms are parallel to the floor. Keep your head, neck, shoulders, and hips aligned. Exhale and push up, back to the starting position, by straightening your elbows.

➤ *Variations* For an easier intensity, perform the exercise with both knees on the floor.

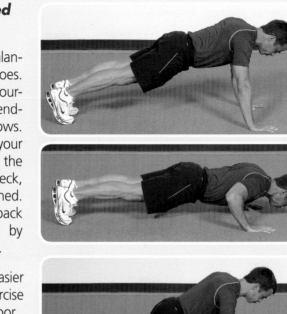

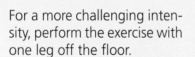

For a more challenging intensity, perform the exercise with one leg off the floor.

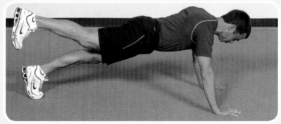

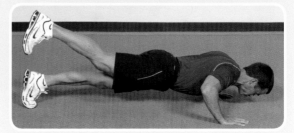

ABDOMINAL CRUNCH

➢ *Muscle Group Worked*
Abdominals

➢ *Execution*   Start by lying down with your knees bent and your feet flat on the floor. Place your hands above your thighs and raise your head, neck, and shoulders slightly off the floor while keeping your low back on the floor. Then lift your shoulders higher off the floor by contracting your abdominal muscles. Slowly lower to the starting position without resting your back on the floor.

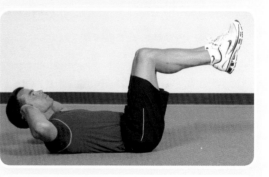

➢ *Variation*   For a more challenging intensity, perform the exercise with your hands at your ears and both feet off the floor, bending your knees at a 90-degree angle.

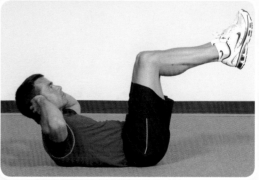

BODY WEIGHT

STEP-UP

> ***Muscle Group Worked***
Legs

> ***Execution*** Start by stepping with one foot onto a chair. Lift yourself onto the chair using the same leg. Lower your foot back to the floor, then switch legs.

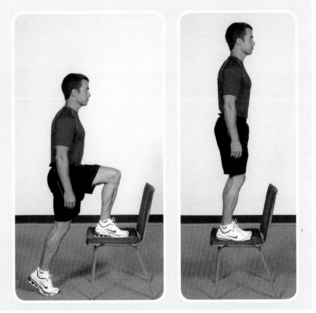

SQUAT

> ***Muscle Group Worked*** Legs

> ***Execution*** Start with your feet shoulder-width apart. Inhale, then lower your body into a sitting position. Your back should be straight and your chest up. Keep your weight on your heels and make sure to keep your knees over your ankles. Exhale as you straighten your legs and return to the starting position.

> ***Variation*** For a more challenging intensity, perform the exercise with one leg (photo on right).

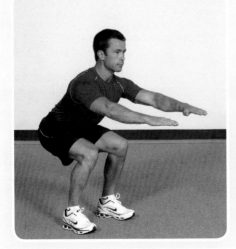
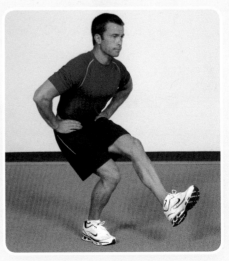

TRICEPS DIP

▷ **Muscle Group Worked** Triceps

▷ **Execution** Start with the palms of your hands on the edge of a chair or box and your feet straight out in front of you. Slowly lower your body toward the floor by bending your arms at the elbow joints. Keep your hips close to the chair or box and try not to use your legs. Push yourself back up to the starting position by straightening your elbows.

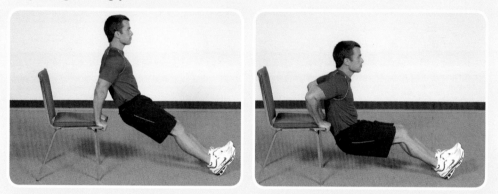

▷ **Variations** For an easier intensity, place your feet flat on the floor and bend your knees.

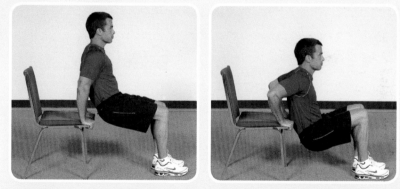

For a more challenging intensity, lift one leg up off the floor and use the other for balance.

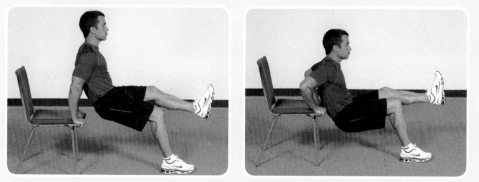

BODY WEIGHT

PLANK

> *Muscle Group Worked*   Core

> *Execution*   Start by placing your forearms and toes on the floor. Slowly push your body up off the floor and balance on your forearms and toes. At the same time, contract your abdominal muscles and keep your head, neck, and shoulders aligned. Hold this position for 30 seconds.

> *Variations*   For an easier intensity, balance on your forearms and knees.

For a more challenging intensity, lift one leg off the floor.

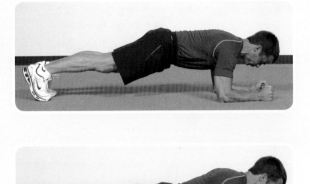

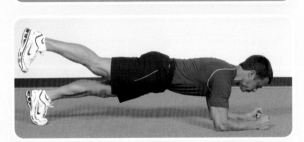

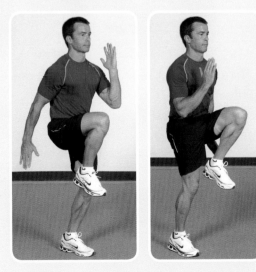

HIGH-KNEES

> *Muscle Group Worked*   Legs

> *Execution*   Start in a standing position with your feet shoulder-width apart. Begin by lifting one knee at a time toward your chest. Lower and repeat with the other leg, as if running in place. This exercise should be performed at a rapid pace.

PUSH–UP AND ROTATION

≫ *Muscle Groups Worked*
Chest and core

≫ *Execution*   Start in the push-up position, then lower your body to the floor. Exhale as you straighten your arms and return to the starting position. As you return to the starting position, rotate your body and lift one arm off the floor. Balance on one arm and both legs in a side plank position. Rotate back to the starting position and repeat for the opposite side.

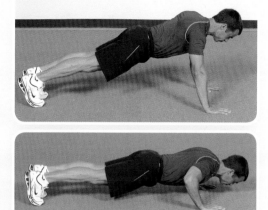

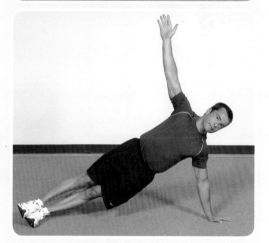

≫ *Variation*   For an easier intensity, perform this exercise on your knees (below).

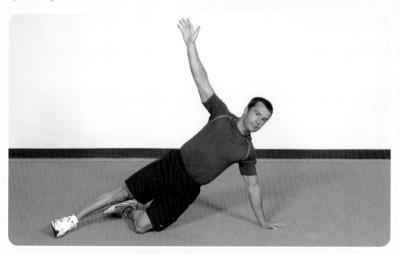

BODY WEIGHT

SIDE PLANK

> *Muscle Group Worked*   Core

> *Execution*   Start by lying on your side. Lift your hips off the floor by contracting your abdominal muscles and balancing on your forearms and feet. Keep your body straight and your hips up toward the ceiling. Hold this position for 30 seconds, then repeat for the other side.

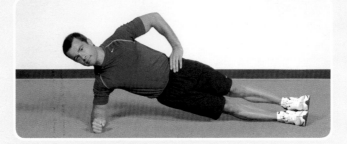

> *Variations*   For an easier intensity, place your bottom knee on the ground.

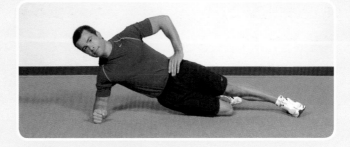

For a more challenging intensity, lift your top leg and hold.

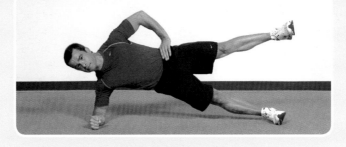

CHEST PRESS WITH RESISTANCE BAND

> *Muscle Group Worked*
Chest

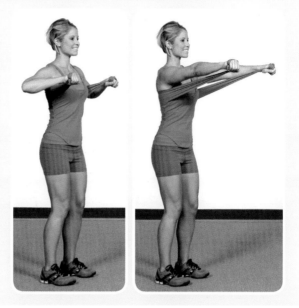

> *Execution* Start with your feet shoulder-width apart, your knees slightly bent, and your back straight. Place the resistance band behind your back and underneath your arms at shoulder-blade height. Hold the ends of the resistance band to create tension. Slowly push your arms out in front of you until they are almost straight, then return to the starting position and repeat.

CHEST FLY WITH RESISTANCE BAND

> *Muscle Group Worked* Chest

> *Execution* Start with your feet shoulder-width apart, your knees slightly bent, and your back straight. Place the resistance band behind your back and on top of your arms at shoulder-blade level. Extend your arms out to your sides

until they are almost straight, holding the ends of the resistance band to create tension. Slowly bring your hands together in front of your body, then return to the starting position.

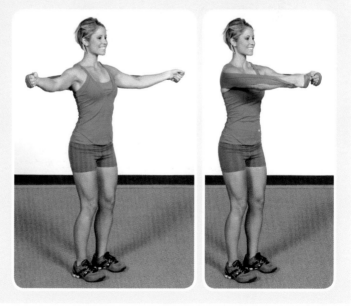

RESISTANCE BANDS

ARM PULL-DOWN WITH RESISTANCE BAND

≫ *Muscle Group Worked*   Back

≫ *Execution*   Start with your feet shoulder-width apart, your knees slightly bent, and your back straight. Hold the resistance band above your head, then slowly pull the band down to your chest while extending your arms to the sides. Squeeze your shoulder blades together and keep your arms almost completely straight. Slowly return to the starting position.

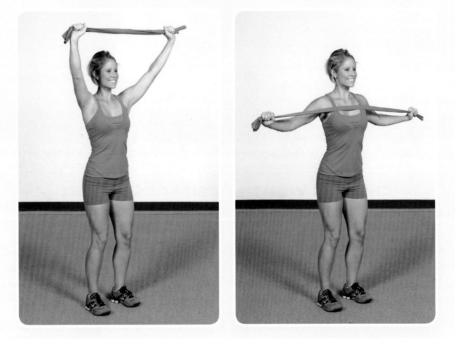

BACK ROW WITH RESISTANCE BAND

▷ ***Muscle Group Worked***   Back

▷ ***Execution***   Start by sitting on the floor with your back straight, your feet directly in front of you, and your knees slightly bent. Place the resistance band around the soles of your feet and firmly grasp each end of the resistance band. Pull the resistance band backward by moving only your elbows and squeezing your shoulder blades together. Slowly return to the starting position.

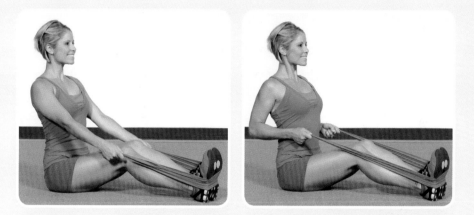

▷ ***Variation***   You can perform this exercise standing up. Place the resistance band underneath one foot, grasp both ends of the resistance band, and keep your back straight and your core tight as you bend over slightly. Pull the resistance band toward your core by moving only your elbows and squeezing your shoulder blades together.

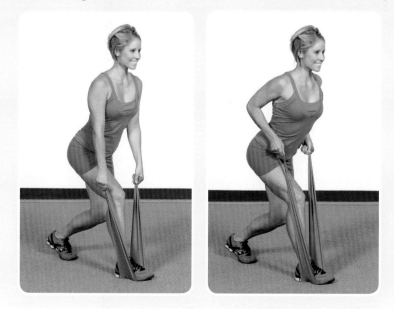

RESISTANCE
BANDS

SQUAT WITH RESISTANCE BAND

> *Muscle Group Worked*   Legs

> *Execution*   Start by laying the resistance band on the floor and stepping on it with both feet. Place your feet about shoulder-width apart and hold both ends of the resistance band. Bend your knees and squat down into a sitting position, keeping your chest up and your weight on your heels. Lower yourself only as far as your knees will comfortably bend. Wrap your hands around the resistance band to take up the slack, then bring your hands to shoulder height. Slowly stand up and return to the starting position.

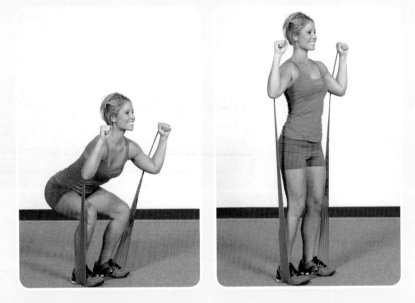

> *Variations*   For an easier intensity, either do not use the resistance band, or bring your hands down by your side.

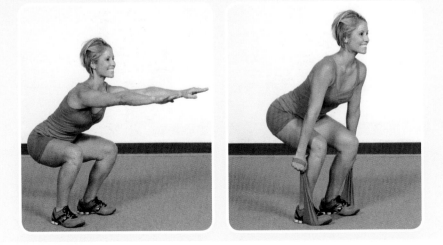

SPLIT SQUAT WITH RESISTANCE BAND

▷ *Muscle Group Worked*   Legs

▷ *Execution*   Start by laying the resistance band on the floor and stepping on it with one foot. Bring your other leg behind you and let your back heel come up off the floor. Slowly drop your back knee toward the ground, allowing your front knee to bend at the same time. Wrap your hands around the resistance band to take up the slack. Keep your upper body straight at all times, do not lean forward, and do not let your knees extend over past your front toes. Return slowly to the starting position and repeat with the other leg.

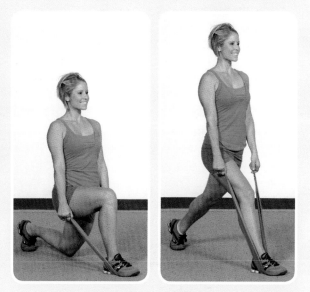

▷ *Variation*   For a more challenging intensity, place the resistance band under your front foot. When you bend your knees, take up the slack of the resistance band by wrapping your hands around the ends of the band and bringing your hands to shoulder level. Continue with the same movement as previously stated.

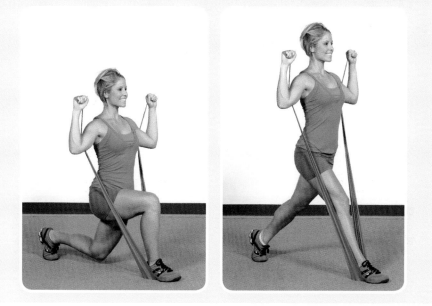

RESISTANCE BANDS

RESISTANCE BANDS

SHOULDER PRESS WITH RESISTANCE BAND

> **Muscle Group Worked**   Shoulders

> **Execution** Start by laying the resistance band on the floor, then stepping on it with both feet. Stand with your feet shoulder-width apart and firmly grasp both ends of the resistance band. Holding each end of the band, wrap the band once around each hand. Bring both hands up to shoulder height and bend your elbows at a 90-degree angle. This is the starting position. Straighten your arms by pressing upward and bringing your hands above your head. Slowly bring your arms back to the starting position.

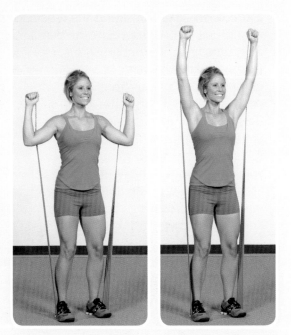

> **Variation**   For an easier intensity, place only one foot on the resistance band and bring the other in front of your body.

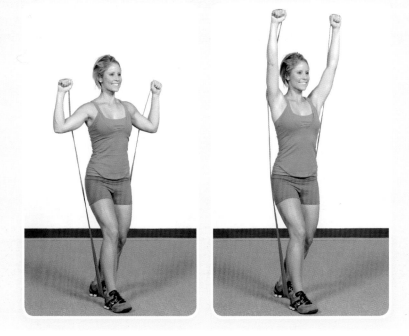

LATERAL RAISE WITH RESISTANCE BAND

➤ *Muscle Group Worked*   Shoulders

➤ *Execution*   Start by laying the resistance band on the floor and stepping on it with both feet. Stand with your feet shoulder-width apart and your knees slightly bent, and firmly grasp both ends of the resistance band. Holding each end of the band, wrap the band once around each hand. With your arms slightly bent and your palms facing down, raise both arms simultaneously out to your sides, no higher than shoulder level. Slowly return to the starting position.

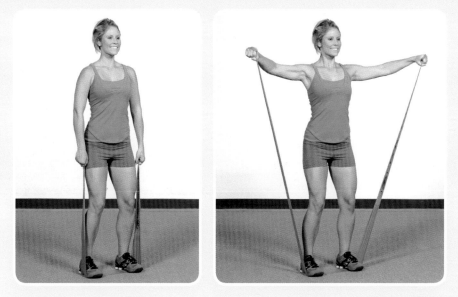

➤ *Variation*   For an easier intensity, take one foot off of the resistance band.

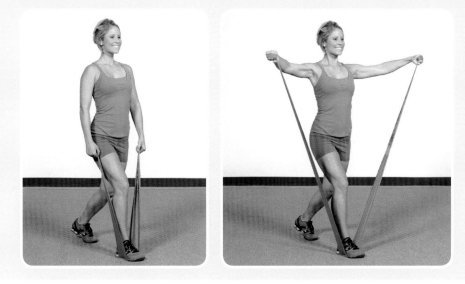

RESISTANCE BANDS

BICEPS CURL WITH RESISTANCE BAND

≫ **Muscle Group Worked**   Biceps

≫ **Execution**   Start by laying the resistance band on the floor and stepping on it with both feet. Stand with your feet shoulder-width apart and your knees slightly bent, and firmly grasp both ends of the resistance band. Wrap the band one or more times around each hand. Raise both of your arms in front of your body, bending your arms at the elbows. Keep your wrists straight and your elbows against your sides. Slowly return to the starting position.

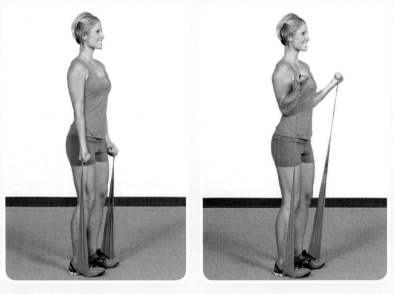

≫ **Variation**   For an easier intensity, step on the resistance band with one foot instead of both feet.

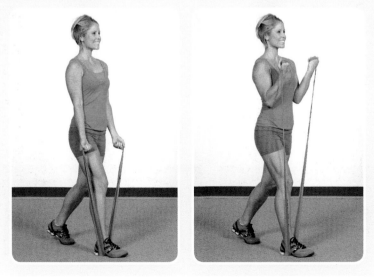

RESISTANCE BANDS

TRICEPS EXTENSION WITH RESISTANCE BAND

> *Muscle Group Worked* Triceps

> *Execution* Start by laying the resistance band on the floor and stepping on it with both feet. Stand with your feet shoulder-width apart and your knees slightly bent and firmly grasp both ends of the resistance band. Holding each end of the band, wrap the band once around each hand. Bring your hands behind your head with your elbows close to your ears. Push your arms straight up, using your triceps, while keeping your elbows close to your ears. Slowly return to the starting position.

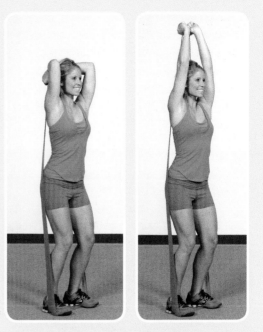

RESISTANCE BANDS

> *Variations* For an easier intensity, perform the same exercise with one foot in the middle of the resistance band or hold only one end of the resistance band.

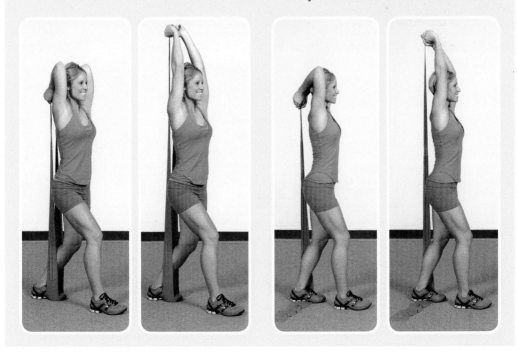

ABDOMINAL CRUNCH WITH RESISTANCE BAND

≫ *Muscle Group Worked* Abdominals

≫ *Execution* Start by lying on your back with your feet resting in the middle of the resistance band and your hands holding the band at both ends. Place your hands behind your head and keep your chin up. Keep your feet flat on the floor at a 45-degree angle. Lift your head, neck, and shoulders off the floor. Slowly crunch your body toward your knees until your lower back is almost ready to lift off the floor. Keep your chin off of your chest and look up. Hold at the top for 1 second, then slowly lower to the starting position.

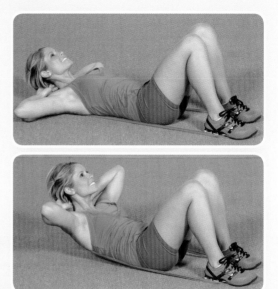

REVERSE LOW-BACK EXTENSION WITH RESISTANCE BAND

≫ *Muscle Group Worked* Low back

≫ *Execution* Starting on your hands and knees, wrap the resistance band around the sole of your right foot and grasp the ends of the resistance band. Keeping your neck and back straight, extend your right leg backward against the band until your leg is parallel to the floor. Slowly return to the starting position. Repeat with your other leg.

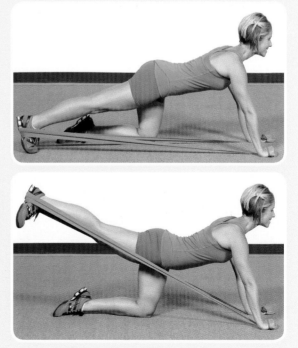

DUMBBELL CHEST PRESS ON STABILITY BALL

➢ *Muscle Group Worked* Chest

➢ *Execution* Holding a dumbbell in each hand, start in a seated position on the ball. Slowly walk your feet out until your head and shoulders are supported by the ball. Place your feet shoulder-width apart to create stability. Contract your core and bring your hands to chest level with your palms facing forward. Then press your arms upward until your hands are directly above your chest and your arms are almost completely straight. Once you have reached the top position, bring the dumbbells down to the starting position.

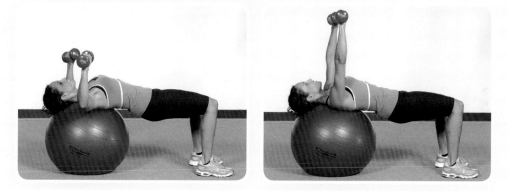

DUMBBELL CHEST FLY ON STABILITY BALL

➢ *Muscle Group Worked* Chest

➢ *Execution* Holding a dumbbell in each hand, start in a seated position on the ball. Slowly walk your feet out until your head and shoulders are supported by the ball. Place your feet shoulder-width apart to create stability. Contract your core and place your arms above your chest with your palms facing one another. Slowly lower your arms to the sides with your elbows slightly bent. Stop when your upper arms are parallel to the floor. Return to the starting position.

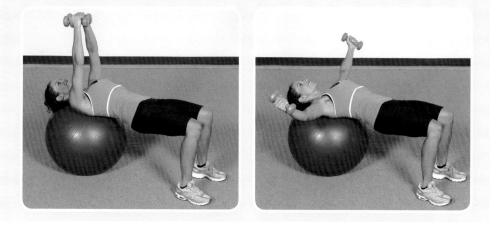

STABILITY BALLS

STABILITY BALLS

DUMBBELL PULLOVER ON STABILITY BALL

▷ *Muscle Group Worked*
Back

▷ *Execution* Starting in a seated position on the ball, slowly walk your feet out until your head and shoulders are supported by the ball. Place your feet shoulder-width apart to create stability. Hold the dumbbell with both of your hands, bring your arms above your head, and slightly bend your arms at the elbows. Lower the dumbbell behind your head while maintaining a slight bend at your elbows. Stop when your arms are parallel with the floor or when you feel a stretch in your upper back. Slowly bring the dumbbell back to the starting position.

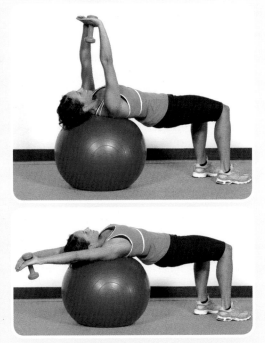

DUMBBELL SINGLE-ARM ROW ON STABILITY BALL

▷ *Muscle Group Worked* Back

▷ *Execution* Start in a standing position. Place one knee on top of the ball while maintaining balance with your other foot on the floor. Hold a dumbbell in one hand and place the other hand on the ball. Move the elbow of the arm holding the dumbbell upward. You should feel your shoulder blades squeeze together. Make sure to keep your back straight and aligned with your shoulders and hips. Slowly lower the dumbbell back to the starting position. Repeat for the other side.

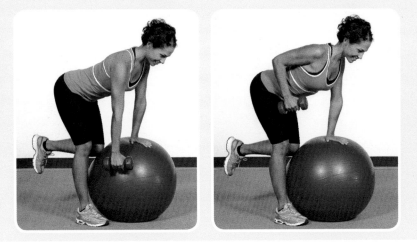

WALL SQUAT WITH STABILITY BALL

> *Muscle Group Worked*
Legs

> *Execution* Stand facing away from a wall. Place the stability ball against the wall at the height of your lower back. Place your feet 12 inches (30 centimeters) in front of your body in a shoulder-width stance and with your toes pointing forward. This exercise can be done with or without dumbbells. Lean into the ball and lower your body until your knees are bent at a 90-degree angle. As you squat, the ball will move to your mid- and upper-back region. Note your feet—your weight should be on your heels, not your toes, and your knees should be aligned with your ankles. Slowly return to the starting position.

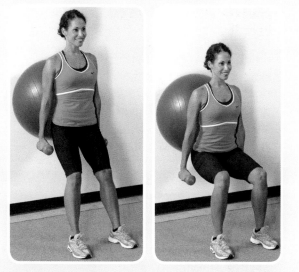

SPLIT SQUAT WITH STABILITY BALL

> *Muscle Group Worked* Legs

> *Execution* Stand in front of your ball and place one foot on top of the ball while resting a hand on the wall for support (or hold a dumbbell in each hand). Shuffle your other foot forward and shift your weight onto this support leg. Your front foot should point forward, and your knee should stay directly above your ankle. Contract your core. Drop your hips until the front leg is bent at a 90-degree angle. Make sure that the knee of your front leg is not beyond your toes—if it is, your stance is too short, and you need to place your foot farther in front of you. Slowly return to the starting position.

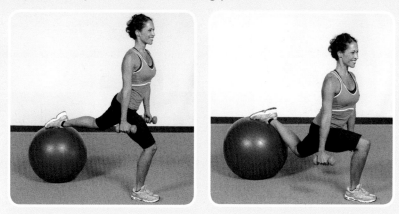

DUMBBELL SHOULDER PRESS ON STABILITY BALL

> ▷ **Muscle Group Worked**   Shoulders

> ▷ **Execution** Holding a dumbbell in each hand, start in a seated position on the ball. Place your feet shoulder-width apart to create stability. Bring your hands up to shoulder height with your palms facing forward. Press your arms straight above your head. Make sure to maintain good posture with a straight back. Slowly lower to the starting position, making sure that your elbows do not drop below shoulder height.

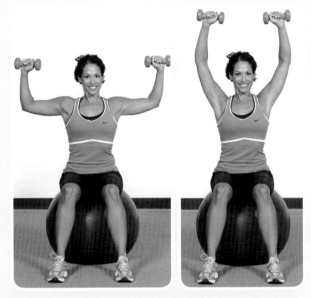

DUMBBELL LATERAL RAISE ON STABILITY BALL

> ▷ **Muscle Group Worked**   Shoulders

> ▷ **Execution**   Start in a seated position on the ball with arms down by your sides, holding a dumbbell in each hand. Raise your arms out to the sides, no higher than shoulder height, with your elbows slightly bent and your palms facing down. Slowly return to the starting position.

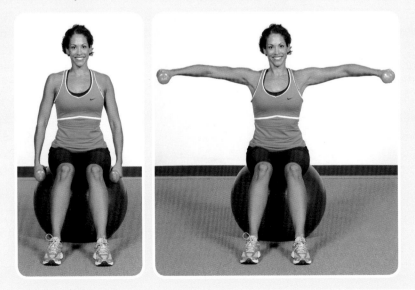

DUMBBELL BICEPS CURL ON STABILITY BALL

> *Muscle Group Worked* Biceps

> *Execution* Holding a dumbbell in each hand, start in a seated position on the ball. Place your feet shoulder-width apart to create stability. Lower your hands to your sides. Keep your elbows stationary by your sides and curl your forearms up to contract your biceps muscles. Slowly return to the starting position.

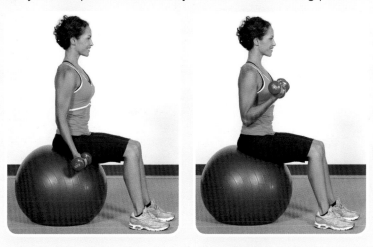

OVERHEAD TRICEPS EXTENSION ON STABILITY BALL

> *Muscle Group Worked* Triceps

> *Execution* Start in a seated position on the ball. Hold one dumbbell in your hands and raise your arms above your head. Keeping your elbows close to your head and in a stationary position, lower the dumbbell behind your head. Slowly return to the starting position.

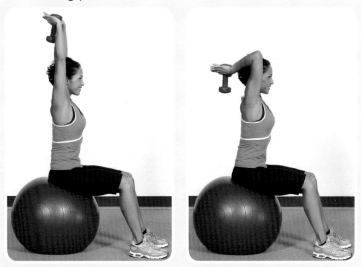

STABILITY BALLS

ABDOMINAL CRUNCH ON STABILITY BALL

⯈ *Muscle Group Worked*   Abdominals

⯈ *Execution*   Start in a seated position on the ball. Slowly walk your feet out until your lower back is supported by the ball. Place your feet shoulder-width apart to create stability. Do not pull your head forward with your hands. Crunch forward by contracting your abdominals, look up, and keep your chin off your chest. Slowly lower to the starting position.

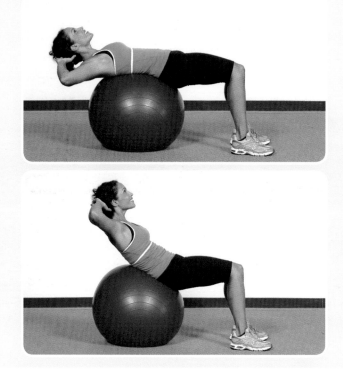

STABILITY BALLS

LOW-BACK EXTENSION ON STABILITY BALL

▷ **Muscle Group Worked**   Low back

▷ **Execution**   Start by kneeling behind the stability ball and resting your abdomen on top of it. Place your hands on the floor and slowly walk your arms out until your hips and abdomen are supported by the ball. Place your forearms on the ground, using them for support, then raise your legs until your body is fully extended and your back is straight. Slowly return to the starting position.

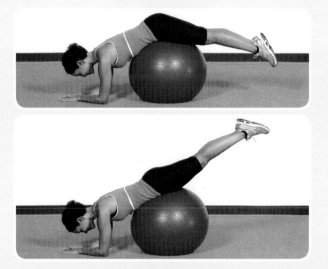

▷ **Variation**   Start by kneeling behind the stability ball and resting your abdomen on top of it. Straighten your legs. Place your hands behind your head and lower your head toward the front of the stability ball, using your knees for support and balance. Raise your torso until you feel tightness in your lower back. Be sure not to overextend your low back.

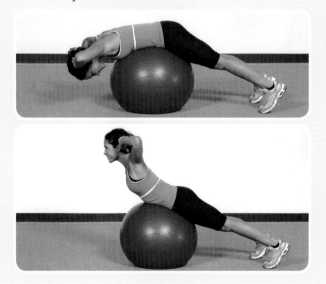

BARBELL BENCH PRESS

≫ *Muscle Group Worked*   Chest

≫ *Execution*   Lie down on the bench and grip the barbell with your hands just wider than shoulder-width apart. Remove the bar from the rack and slowly lower the bar toward your chest. Once the bar has reached your chest, slowly raise it back to the starting position. Rerack the bar after you have finished a complete set.

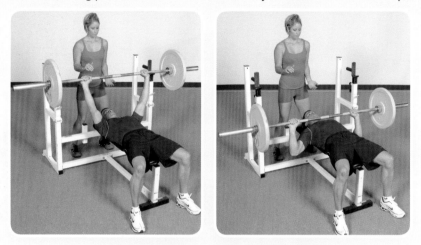

DUMBBELL INCLINE FLY

≫ *Muscle Group Worked*   Chest

≫ *Execution*   Start by adjusting the bench to a 45-degree angle. Holding a dumbbell in each hand, lie on the bench and place your feet on the floor. Contract your core and bring your arms above your chest with your palms facing each other. Slowly lower your arms to your sides with your elbows slightly bent. Stop when your upper arms are parallel to the floor. Return to the starting position.

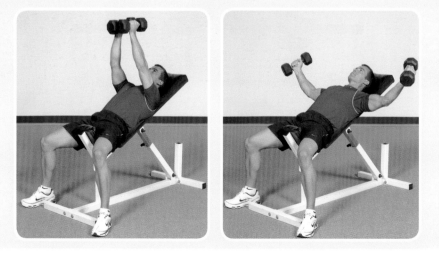

FREE WEIGHTS

WIDE-GRIP CHIN-UP

≫ *Muscle Group Worked* Back

≫ *Execution* Grab the outside handles of a pull-up bar or machine. Pull yourself up toward the bar, leading with your chest and squeezing your shoulder blades together. Slowly return to the starting position.

≫ *Variations* Perform the same exercise using an assisted-lift pull-up machine (bottom left), or use a close grip (bottom right).

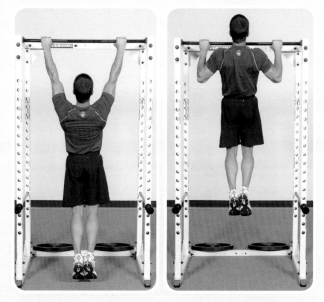

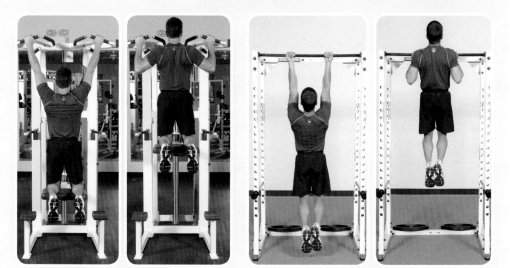

FREE WEIGHTS

BARBELL BENT-OVER ROW

> *Muscle Group Worked* Back

> *Execution*   Stand with your feet shoulder-width apart and your knees slightly bent. Bend over at your hips while keeping your back straight and your shoulders back. Grip the bar with your hands shoulder-width apart. Raise the bar up toward your abdominal area by bringing your elbows behind your back and squeezing your shoulder blades together. Slowly return to the starting position.

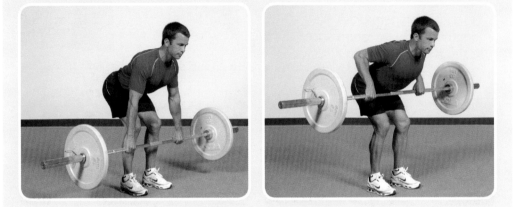

BARBELL SQUAT

> *Muscle Group Worked*   Legs

> *Execution*   Start with your feet shoulder-width apart and your knees slightly bent. Place the barbell across your back and shoulders (make sure to grip the bar firmly). Then lower yourself toward the floor by bending at your knee and hip joints. Hold the barbell steady across your back and shoulders. Keep your chest up and your back straight. Also make sure to keep the weight on your heels and keep your heels on the floor and your knees over your toes. Slowly return to the starting position.

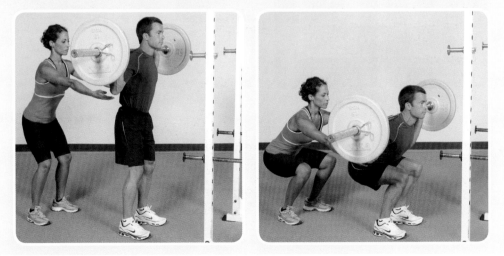

BARBELL STIFF-LEG DEADLIFT

▷ *Muscle Group Worked*   Legs

▷ *Execution*   Standing with your feet shoulder-width apart and your knees slightly bent, hold the barbell in front of you and close to your body. Begin by lowering
the barbell toward the floor, keeping it close to your body. Lower the barbell by
bending at your hips and make sure to keep your back straight and your shoulders
pulled back. Stop when you feel a stretch in the back of your legs or when the
weight has almost reached the floor. Slowly return to the upright starting position.

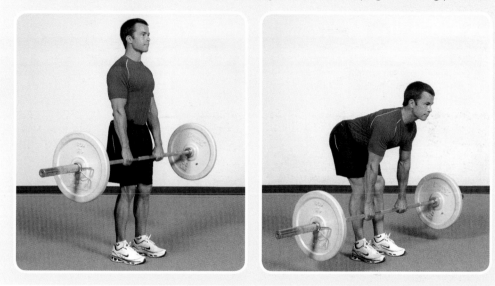

DUMBBELL SHOULDER PRESS

▷ *Muscle Group Worked*
Shoulders

▷ *Execution*   Holding a dumbbell in each hand, start in a
seated position on the bench.
Bend your elbows and bring
your hands to the shoulders
with your palms facing forward. Press your arms straight
above your head. Make sure
to keep your back straight.
Slowly lower to the starting
position, making sure that
your elbows do not drop below shoulder height.

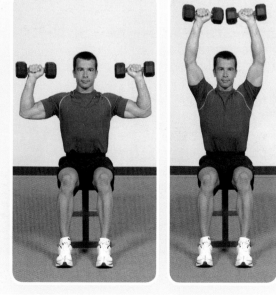

FREE WEIGHTS

BARBELL UPRIGHT ROW

> *Muscle Group Worked*   Shoulders

> *Execution*   Stand with your feet shoulder-width apart and your knees slightly bent and hold the barbell in front of you, gripping it with your hands approximately 6 inches (15 centimeters) apart. Bring the barbell up to your collarbone by leading with your elbows and keeping the bar close to your body. Slowly lower and return to the starting position.

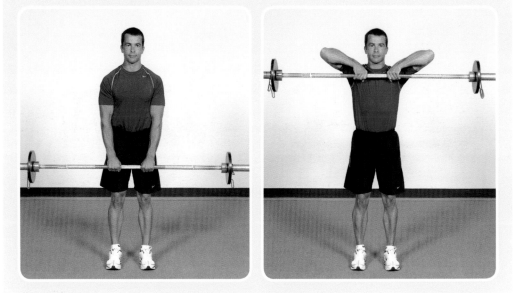

BARBELL BICEPS CURL

> *Muscle Group Worked*
Biceps

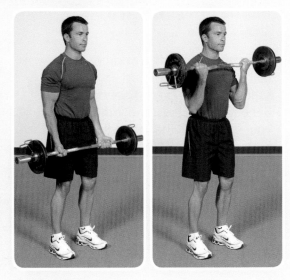

> *Execution*   Stand with your feet shoulder-width apart and your knees slightly bent and hold the barbell in front of you. Keep your elbows stationary by your sides and lift the barbell up toward your chest by contracting your biceps. Slowly return to the starting position.

FREE WEIGHTS

BARBELL TRICEPS EXTENSION

≫ **Muscle Group Worked**   Triceps

≫ **Execution**   Lie flat on the bench. Hold the barbell in your hands and extend your arms over your chest. Lower the barbell toward your head by bending your arms at the elbows (keep your elbows in place as you raise and lower the barbell). Slowly return to the starting position.

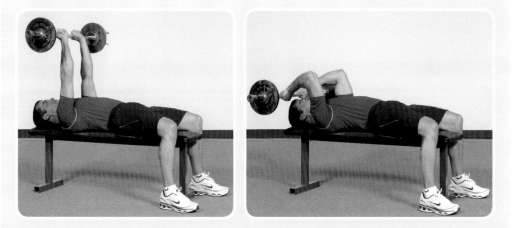

INCLINE BENCH SIT-UP

≫ **Muscle Group Worked**   Abdominals

≫ **Execution**   While lying on the incline bench, hook your feet through the bottom pad. From here, curl yourself up toward your knees by contracting your abdominals; keep your back straight and your chin up.

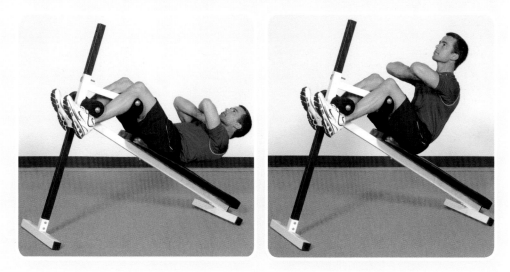

FREE WEIGHTS

LOW-BACK EXTENSION

> *Muscle Group Worked*   Low back

> *Execution*   Start by adjusting the bench apparatus to fit your body. Lower your upper body toward the ground by bending forward at your hips. Place your hands behind your head and raise your upper body by contracting the muscles of your lower back, your glutes, and your hamstrings until your head, neck, and shoulders are aligned.

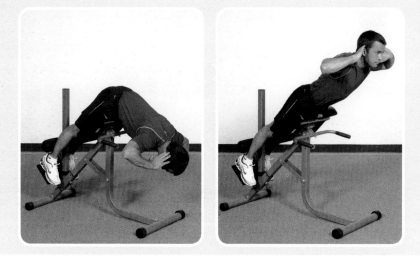

CABLE CHEST PRESS (STAGGERED STANCE)

⟫ *Muscle Group Worked*   Chest

⟫ *Execution*   Stand with your feet approximately 12 inches apart and one in front of the other (i.e., in a staggered stance) and your knees slightly bent. Position the cables on the machine so that the handles are centered at chest height.

Grab both handles and place them to the sides of your chest. Start the exercise by pushing the cables forward in front of your chest until your arms are almost straight. Slowly return to the starting position.

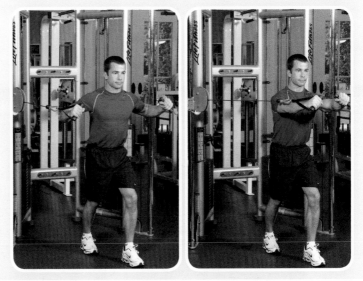

CABLE CHEST FLY (STAGGERED STANCE)

⟫ *Muscle Group Worked*   Chest

⟫ *Execution*   Stand with a staggered stance. Position the cables on the machine so that the handles are centered at chest height. Grab both handles with your palms facing forward and your arms slightly bent. Start by bringing the cables

together so that your hands meet in front of you. Slowly return to the starting position.

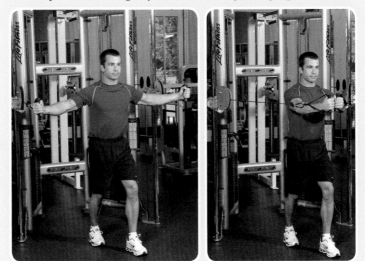

CABLE MACHINES

CABLE DUAL LAT PULL-DOWN

▷ *Muscle Group Worked* Back

▷ *Execution* Position the cables at the machine's top setting. Kneel on the floor or sit on a stability ball with your feet flat on the floor and grasp both handles. Pull the handles down toward your chest, keeping your back straight. As you pull the cables down, squeeze your shoulder blades together. Slowly return to the starting position.

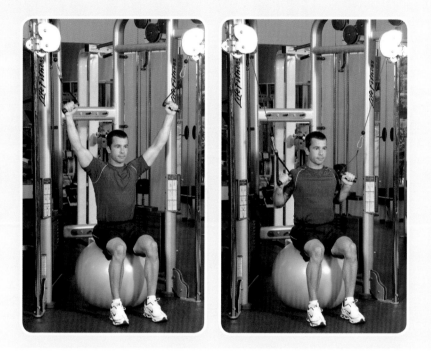

CABLE SINGLE-ARM ROW

≫ *Muscle Group Worked* Back

≫ *Execution* Position the cables at the machine's bottom setting. Stand with your feet in a staggered stance and your knees slightly bent. Hold a cable in one hand and bend over slightly at your hips. Pull the cable backward by squeezing your shoulder blades together and allowing your elbow to go behind your back. Make sure to keep your back straight and aligned with your shoulders and hips. Slowly lower your arm to the starting position. Repeat for the opposite side.

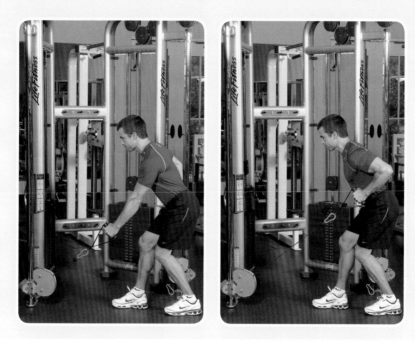

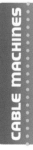

CABLE SQUAT

> **Muscle Group Worked**   Legs

> **Execution**   Position the cables at the machine's bottom setting. Stand with your feet shoulder-width apart and connect the cables to a waist belt. (If you do not have a waist belt, place the cables at the machine's bottom setting and perform the same exercise while holding the cables in your hands.) Lower yourself toward the ground and bend at your knees and hip joints. Keep your chest up and your back straight. Make sure to keep the weight on your heels, your heels on the floor, and your knees over your toes. Slowly return to the starting position.

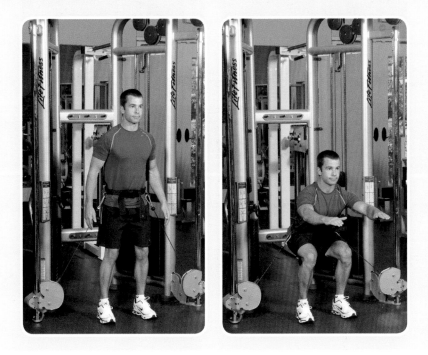

CABLE STEP-UP

▷ *Muscle Group Worked* Legs

▷ *Execution* Position the cables at the machine's bottom setting and connect the cables to a waist belt. (If you do not have a waist belt, place the cables at the machine's bottom setting and perform the same exercise while holding the cables in your hands.) Step with one foot onto the box or onto a stable chair. Use the same leg to lift yourself onto the box. Lower your foot back to the floor, then switch legs.

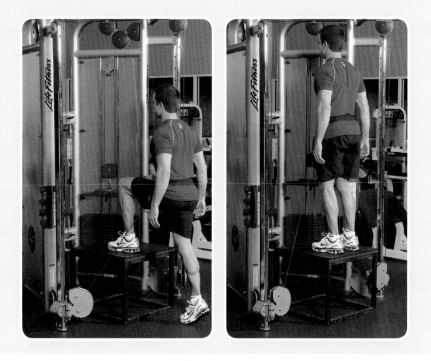

CABLE MACHINES

CABLE DUAL SHOULDER PRESS
(STAGGERED STANCE)

▷ *Muscle Group Worked*   Shoulders

▷ *Execution*   Position the cables at the machine's bottom setting, then grab both handles and bring them to shoulder height with your palms facing forward. Stand with your feet in a staggered stance. (For a more stable position, stand with your feet shoulder-width apart.) Press your arms straight above your head. Slowly lower to the starting position.

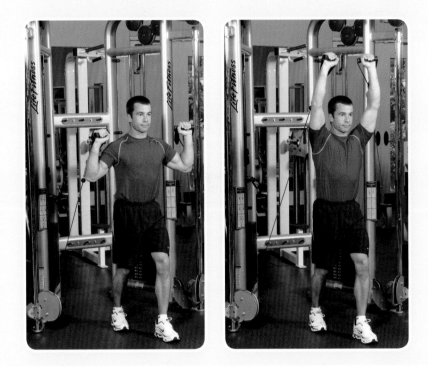

CABLE REVERSE WOOD CHOP

≫ *Muscle Group Worked*   Shoulders

≫ *Execution*   Position the cables at the machine's bottom setting. Grab one cable with both hands and place yourself in a half-squat position. Lift the cable diagonally from a low position to a high position and allow your hips to pivot on the back foot as the motion ends. Slowly return to the starting position.

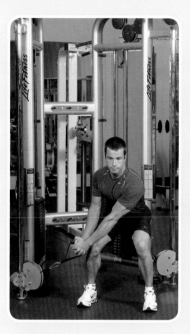
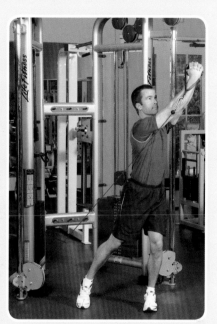

SINGLE-ARM BICEPS CURL WITH CABLE

➤ *Muscle Group Worked* Biceps

➤ *Execution* Position the cables at the machine's bottom setting. Stand with your feet in a staggered stance with your knees slightly bent and grab a cable with one hand. (For a more stable position, stand with your feet shoulder-width apart.) Lower your hand to your side. Keep your elbow stationary and lift the cable by contracting your biceps. Slowly return to the starting position. Repeat for the opposite arm.

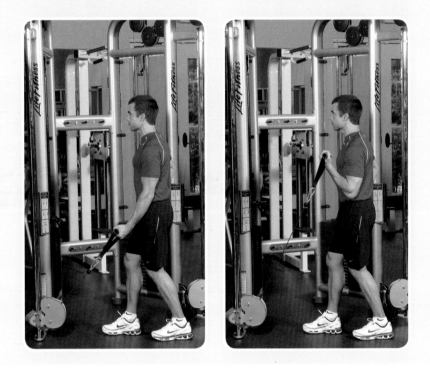

CABLE OVERHEAD TRICEPS EXTENSION

➢ *Muscle Group Worked*   Triceps

➢ *Execution*   Position the cables at the machine's bottom setting. Stand with your feet in a staggered stance with your knees slightly bent and grab the rope attachment with both hands. Bring your hands behind your head with your elbows close to your ears. Extend your arms straight up, using your triceps and keeping your elbows close to your head. Slowly return to the starting position.

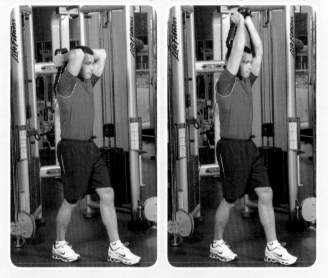

CORE ROTATION WITH CABLE

➢ *Muscle Group Worked*   Core

➢ *Execution*   Position the cables on the machine so that the handles are centered at chest height. Stand with your feet shoulder-width apart with your knees slightly bent and grab one cable with both hands. Keeping your arms straight, pull the cable across your body by rotating your torso. Keep your abdominals tight and your hips stationary. Slowly return to the starting position.

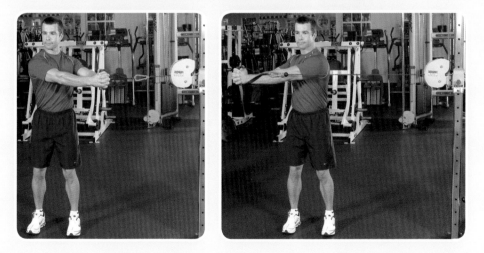

CABLE MACHINES

PUSH-PULL

▷ *Muscle Group Worked*   Core

▷ *Execution*   Position the cables on the machine so that the handles are centered at chest height. Position yourself with one cable in front of you and one behind. Stand with your feet in a staggered stance and your knees slightly bent. Grab the cables and push the back cable forward (as in a chest press) and pull the front cable backward (as in a back row). Keep your abdominals tight and your hips stationary. Slowly return to the starting position. Switching arm positions, repeat the exercise.

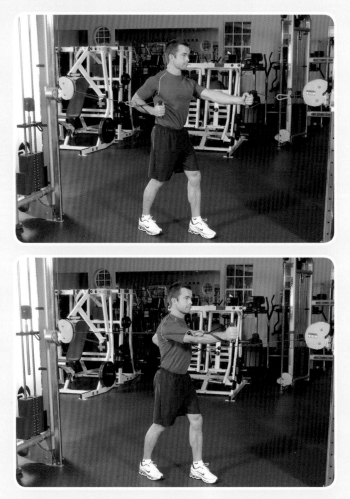

CABLE MACHINES

MACHINE CHEST PRESS

> ### *Muscle Group Worked*   Chest

> ### *Execution*   Sit at the machine and make any necessary adjustments to ensure that your hands are at chest level. Push the handles forward until your arms are almost straight. Make sure to keep your core tight and your back on the bench. Slowly lower to the starting position. You should push forward only with your chest and arms.

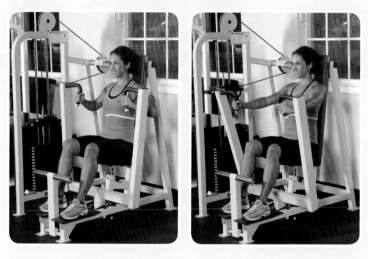

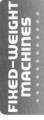

FIXED-WEIGHT MACHINES

PEC DECK

> *Muscle Group Worked* Chest

> *Execution* Sit at the machine and make any necessary adjustments to ensure that your arms are at chest level. Grab both handles and, with your arms slightly bent, bring your hands together in the center. Make sure to keep your core tight and your back on the bench. Slowly return to the starting position.

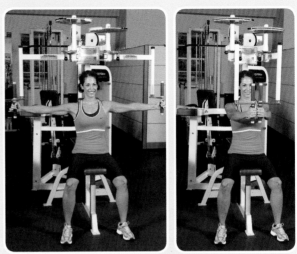

MACHINE LAT PULL-DOWN

> *Muscle Group Worked* Back

> *Execution* Sit at the machine and make any necessary adjustments to ensure that your legs are secured under the knee pad. Grab the straight bar with a wide overhand grip. Relax your shoulders and keep your core tight and your back straight. Lean backward slightly and pull the bar down to the top of your chest. Slowly return to the starting position.

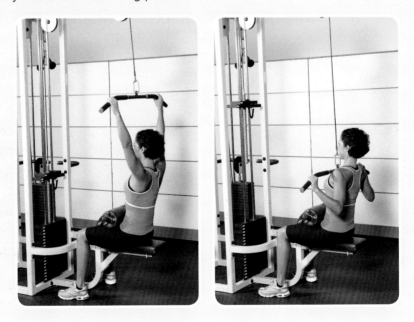

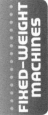

FIXED-WEIGHT MACHINES

MACHINE BACK ROW

▷ *Muscle Group Worked* Back

▷ *Execution* Sit at the machine and make any necessary adjustments to ensure that your chest rests comfortably on the chest pad and that your arms just reach the handles. Grab the handles with an overhand grip. Relax your shoulders and keep your core tight and your back straight. Pull the handles back toward your chest and squeeze your shoulder blades together. Slowly return to the starting position.

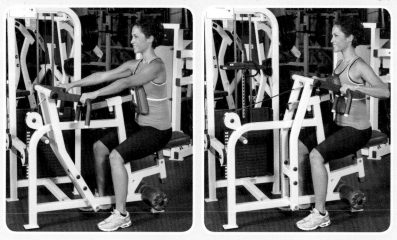

LEG PRESS

▷ *Muscle Group Worked* Legs

▷ *Execution* Sit at the machine and place your feet on the platform. Make any necessary adjustments to ensure that your knees do not extend past your toes and that your feet are shoulder-width apart. Push against the platform with your feet until your legs are almost straight (do not lock your knee joints). This movement will make your seat move backward. Make sure to keep your weight on your heels and your feet flat against the platform. Keep your back flat against the back of the seat and your core tight. Slowly return to the starting position.

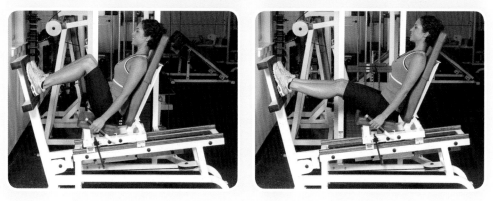

FIXED-WEIGHT MACHINES

PRONE LEG CURL

▷ *MuscleGroupWorked* Legs

▷ **Execution** Lie facedown on the machine and hook your ankles under the ankle pad. Make any necessary adjustments to ensure that your knees are at the pivot point and that the ankle pad does not slip off your legs. Begin by curling your legs up and back toward your glutes. Slowly lower to the starting position.

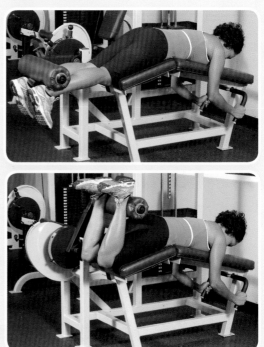

MACHINE SHOULDER PRESS

▷ *Muscle Group Worked*   Shoulders

▷ **Execution**   Sit at the machine and make any necessary adjustments to ensure that the handles rest at your shoulder level. Grab both handles, then push upward until your arms are almost straight. Make sure to keep your back and shoulders flat against the bench and your core tight. Slowly lower to the starting position.

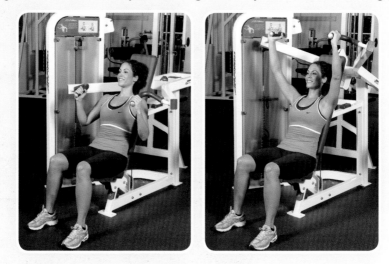

MACHINE LATERAL RAISE

≫ *Muscle Group Worked* Shoulders

≫ *Execution* Sit at the machine and make any necessary adjustments to ensure that your chest is against the chest pad. Place your elbows underneath the arm pads and push the pads out to the sides and up to shoulder height. Make sure to keep your arms in contact with the pads and your core tight. Slowly lower to the starting position.

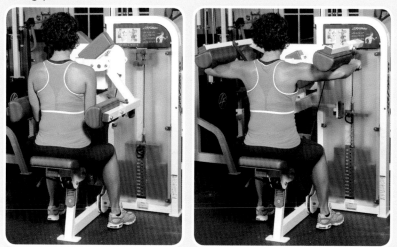

MACHINE BICEPS CURL

≫ *Muscle Group Worked* Biceps

≫ *Execution* Sit at the machine and make any necessary adjustments to ensure that your arms are placed comfortably on the pad and that your elbows are at the pivot point. Grab both handles, then curl the bar up toward your chest while keeping your elbows secure on the pad. Slowly return to the starting position.

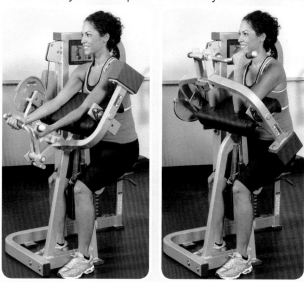

FIXED-WEIGHT MACHINES

MACHINE TRICEPS EXTENSION

> ***Muscle Group Worked***   Triceps

> ***Execution***   Sit at the machine and make any necessary adjustments to ensure that your arms are placed comfortably on the pad and that your elbows are at the pivot point. Grab both handles and push the bar down until your arms are almost straight; keep your elbows secure on the pad. Slowly return to the starting position.

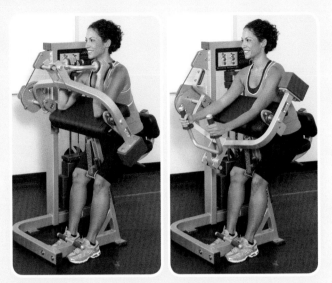

MACHINE ABDOMINAL CRUNCH

> ***Muscle Group Worked***   Abdominals

> ***Execution***   Sit at the machine and make any necessary adjustments to ensure that your chest is placed comfortably on the chest pad. Curl your torso, bringing the pad down to your knees, by contracting your abdominals. Make sure to keep your core tight and use only your abdominals, not your arms. Slowly return to the starting position.

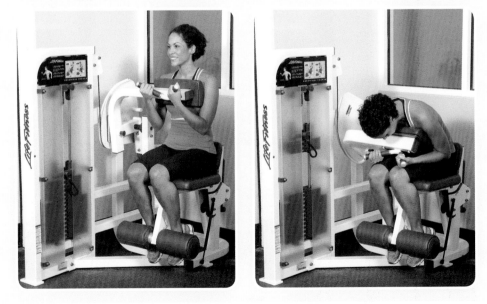

MACHINE LOW-BACK EXTENSION

> **Muscle Group Worked**   Low back

> **Execution**

Sit at the machine and make any necessary adjustments to ensure your hips are at the pivot point. Push the pad backward by extending your lower back. Make sure to keep your core tight. Slowly return to the starting position.

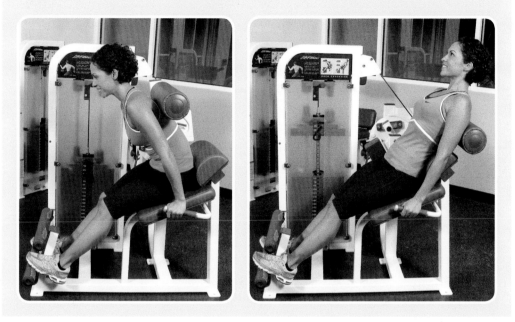

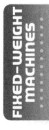

FIXED-WEIGHT MACHINES

PREPARING MENTALLY AND PHYSICALLY

You are about to move from a stage of thinking about physical activity to doing it. This is a critical time, and you need to prepare yourself mentally and emotionally in order to enhance your chances of sticking with it and thus achieving your long-term goals. Here are some thoughts for you to ponder as you get ready to begin.

• Start your program slowly; if you err, do so on the side of caution. If you haven't exercised in some time, choose mild or moderate levels of physical activity. We also suggest that you limit yourself to a maximum of 5 days of activity per week at first, with no individual workout going longer than 45 minutes. As you progress, you can increase at a pace that works for you.

• Be sure to warm up and cool down in order to take care of your body before and after exercise.

• Think of your new plan as one that will help you carry out a journey toward better health, increased fitness, and a higher energy level. This journey begins with a few small steps. You need to be in this for the long haul, so don't expect instant gratification.

• To help spur yourself on each week, keep reading and learning about the energy-related benefits of physical activity.

• Think of each session of physical activity as making a deposit in the bank. It will take some time to grow into a healthier you, but each day of implementing your plan increases your positive balance in the health bank.

• Recognize the difference between pain and discomfort. If you feel a burn during activity or find yourself out of breath or fatigued, it is okay; in fact, it is to be expected. But if you feel a sharp pain, a stinging sensation, lightheadedness, muscle tightness, or a pull—stop what you are doing and reevaluate. You may need to rest, apply ice to reduce swelling, or even get a diagnosis from a professional.

• Try to raise your emotional energy before you begin activity by focusing on your goals, not on the time. Listen to your favorite energizing music if that is an option, look for enjoyment in your surroundings, interact with activity partners, and use positive self-talk to keep your motivation high. Here are some examples.

  • This is precious time, so use it wisely.
  • I'm doing something good for myself.
  • My kids would be proud of me.
  • I'm finally doing it—not just talking.
  • Can't wait to see my spouse's face.

- Relax and enjoy the challenge.
- Don't forget to breathe.
- If I work out hard today, the next day will be easier.
- My skills are improving every time I play.
- A step at a time, a day at a time—and have *fun.*

If negative self-talk crops up, just say *stop* and substitute a positive phrase instead. Besides readying your attitude for physical activity, you also need to fuel your body before, during, and after activity. Here are some tips to get you going and keep you in the game.

- Drink extra fluid before, during, and after exercise. Diluted sports drinks (one part sports drink, one part water) are an excellent choice. If you are active in hot, humid weather, increase your fluid intake considerably because you'll lose plenty through perspiration. As a guide, aim to drink 8 ounces (0.24 liters) of water every 15 minutes during exercise. After exercise, drink 16 ounces (0.47 liters) of water for every pound of body weight lost during exercise. (We recommend that you weigh yourself before and after exercise if you expect to sweat a lot.)

- Eat at least a snack before you exercise. If you choose an early morning workout time and go without breakfast, you may end up burning your own muscle for energy! Your body will feel sluggish, starved, and lacking in energy.

TIPS for High Energy

- Work on your breathing techniques in order to optimize your performance and enjoyment of physical activity.
- Develop a sound routine for warming up and cooling down, and *always* use it. It's fine to add some variety as long as you follow the anatomical principles.
- Study the principles of resistance training in order to maximize muscular strength and endurance training.
- Vary your methods and equipment for strength training in order to keep things fresh, make working out convenient (i.e., use the opportunities at hand), and benefit from the differing virtues of various types of training.
- Consciously adjust your attitude by cultivating positive thoughts and feelings that are energizing.
- Add fuel by eating and drinking before, during, and after physical activity.

A small glass of juice or milk is all it takes to prevent this problem; you can have breakfast after the workout.

- Unless your activity is extremely long, you probably don't need to eat during it, but you do need to replenish your energy stores within 30 minutes after the activity. Your muscles need the fuel replacement, and your body systems overall need the fluid replacement. Half of an energy bar and plenty of water will typically work just fine. Have your next main meal within 2 hours of the workout.

CHAPTER 10

MEASURING SUCCESS

Once you implement your plan for increasing your personal energy through sports and physical activity, it is critical to measure your success accurately. In some cases, you'll be pleasantly surprised by the progress you make; at other times, you may be disappointed. But no matter the outcome, keeping a record is absolutely essential in order to get factual feedback about how you are doing. We suggest that you measure your progress in four ways.

- Evaluate your progress toward achieving your *goals.*
- Keep a *weekly log* of physical activity you have performed.
- Keep a *performance journal* of your thoughts and feelings.
- Conduct a *retest* (identical to your initial fitness test) to evaluate your cardiorespiratory fitness, muscular fitness, flexibility, and body composition.

We cover all of these approaches in greater detail in this chapter. Thus, after reading the chapter, you will have a strategy for ensuring long-term success with your personal prescription for increasing your physical energy.

IDENTIFYING YOUR PERSONAL MISSION AND GOALS

It is important to take a step back and consider your overall mission and your specific goals for increased personal energy. Let's look first at your overall mission for change. What is it that you are trying to accomplish? Here are some possible answers.

- To create more personal energy so that I can consistently perform at a higher level at work
- To create more personal energy so that when I am not working I will have the energy to fully engage with my loved ones
- To feel more confident in my physical being, look better, feel more alive, and have more energy to face each day

- To become healthier through physical activity and enlarge my circle of friends

These simple statements are clear, focused, and expressive of a desired outcome. If you like, feel free to adopt one of these statements, or to combine ideas expressed in them, but, however you arrive at it, your personal mission should be defined in the end by *your* dream or vision. Of course, we think that based on what you have read so far, this mission statement should include some mention of how you plan to create more personal energy or manage it better.

Write your personal mission statement for developing personal energy here:

_____

_____

Now, let's move on to the next level of planning through *setting goals.* To be helpful, a goal should be realistic, specific, and geared to a set period of time in which it will be achieved.

Realistic means that your proposed actions have a reasonable chance of success. For example, if you were to set a goal of exercising every day for 2 hours, it is unlikely that you would find the time or that your body would tolerate that duration of exertion if you have been inactive.

Specificity in a goal is crucial to evaluating success. A vague goal is impossible to measure. For example, the goal "improve my fitness level" is just too vague. Saying that you plan to eat better is equally unspecific. A better goal would be to improve your muscular fitness by performing 30 minutes of strength training twice a week for the next 6 weeks. This goal is specific and requires only that you exert effort to achieve it.

Tying a goal to a time line implies a sense of importance, urgency, and commitment. Think in terms of weekly and monthly intervals in order to evaluate your progress and make adjustments in your plan.

Finally, test your goals to confirm that the number one requirement for you to be successful in pursuing it is simply to invest energy and effort. If your personal program is well thought out, you should be able to focus on your own actions of investing effort rather than rely on outside factors such as other people, weather, or work to ensure your success. Only you can make a decision to invest your energy in the plan and be responsible for following through.

Here are some sample goals that you can use as models in developing your own:

- To increase my intake of water by carrying it with me and sipping it throughout the day
- To plan my physical activity for the week ahead on Sundays and follow the plan for the week

- To make a 2-week plan for physical activity, keep a daily record of achievement, and adjust my plan before the next 2-week period
- To share my commitment with my spouse and children and ask for their help by grading my performance daily
- To add two snacks to my food intake daily and reduce the size of my portions to five handfuls each meal for the next month
- To plan and carry out a schedule for 2 weeks that ensures 7 hours of sleep every night with no exceptions (even on weekends)
- To allocate at least 1 hour each day for relaxation and recreation away from my job, even if it means rising earlier each morning

Write your personal goals here:

_____

_____

_____

_____

_____

RECORDING YOUR ACTIVITY

We presented a sample physical activity schedule in figure 8.1 on page 95. As you review that sample now, notice that for each day we ask you simply to make a quick note of the activity or activities you performed, their duration, and their intensity.

We also suggest that you record a score from 1 to 5 that indicates whether you achieved your goals for that day (5 indicates a full yes). The last column calls for a check mark if you had fun that day. It is up to you to define what fun means to you in this context based on your reading of chapter 6.

For this activity log to be effective, you need to complete it each day so that you keep an accurate record to review at the end of each week. If you don't have a clear record of what you've done, it will be impossible to make smart plans for future weeks.

You can expand your physical activity log to address other specific goals that you have listed. For example, you might add a category about food and use headings along these lines: Ate Breakfast, Ate Two Snacks, Used Portion Control, Stayed Hydrated. You could then put a check mark under headings for which you fulfilled the goal that day. Other possible topics to address in your log include sleep, rest and recovery goals, deep breathing, and relaxation time with spouse or family.

RECORDING YOUR THOUGHTS AND FEELINGS

We suggest that you purchase a blank notebook to use as a personal journal in which you record your thoughts and feelings about your performance each day. There are no rules for this journal except to record the date and write a few sentences about your experience in pursuing your activities to increase your personal energy. You might comment on your sleep, food intake, water intake, breathing, and physical activity, concentrating on what you thought or felt about them. This is not the place to be specific about repetitions performed, time spent, or distance covered, but rather to express your thoughts and feelings about your performance that day.

Here is a sample journal entry:

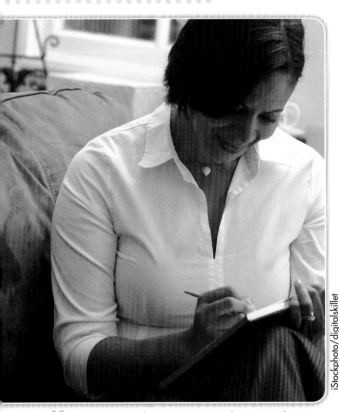

iStockphoto/digitalskillet

Keep a personal exercise journal to record your thoughts and feelings.

Today was a great day! I planned my physical activity, was careful in my warm-up and cool-down, and the time just flew by as I was walking. During the walk, I gradually relaxed from the day's pressures and focused on the promise of spring in the air. By the time I finished, I had worked up a good sweat and felt loose and energized. In fact, I probably could have kept going for another 30 minutes. Oh, I also ate my two snacks today and felt less hungry at meals. I'm making some progress. I feel like I'm finally beginning to make time for me!

We like the idea of using a dedicated notebook for this journal, but if you use a daily planner it could substitute nicely if you write your notes in a special section. You might even want to record your thoughts on a computer or portable electronic device if that is more convenient for you. The point is to just do it somehow, so that you can refer back to your record at the end of the week as you look toward the next week.

Why record your thoughts and feelings? Taking the time to write in your journal forces you to be aware of your progress on a regular basis. It increases your awareness of what worked and what didn't, what felt good and what didn't, what you enjoyed and what was not fun; as a result, you can make smarter, more informed decisions about each week's activity plan. For instance, if you reluctantly tried a new cardio machine because your usual machine was unavailable and you really enjoyed the change, make a note of this experience. In addition, the very act of recording your thoughts and feelings helps you cultivate the self-discipline and commitment that are necessary if you want to establish positive rituals and habits that move you toward your overall goal.

We also know from research in the field of behavioral change that writing about your feelings *soon after* an activity helps imprint the impression in your brain and increases your chance of being able to recall it later. While you may be tempted to simply rely on your memory of your feelings when you reevaluate the impact of your activity program, we're convinced that a documented physical record is a more accurate reflection of your feelings at the time and thus a more powerful motivator.

RETESTING

Success is a powerful driver of motivation, positive thoughts, and feelings, and measuring your progress through retesting can boost your desire to be physically active. It is great to discover that your effort and commitment have paid off; it makes you want to do more. If, on the other hand, you have not made progress, retesting can help you decide on an effective course correction—and it may even make you more determined.

After 6 to 8 weeks, you should replicate the physical testing you performed at the outset. Be sure to make the testing identical to the original test in every way, including location, method, warm-up, trials, and sequence of tests. This approach allows you to make a fair comparison between tests to see if you have made progress.

Progress means success, and any progress you have made, no matter how small, should be welcomed. It means that what you have done has worked. Look at all of your test data carefully and celebrate your successes. For example, has your cardiorespiratory fitness increased, or are you stronger, or can you reach farther? Any of these improvements alone is an indication of success. Perhaps you are just enjoying being physically active more than you thought you would, or maybe you did not miss one planned activity for the last 6 weeks. These too are signs of progress!

If you have made progress, you can continue with the same physical activity program and reasonably expect additional progress. However, we recommend doing no more than 12 weeks of the same program. After 12 weeks, you should consider adding some variety. Your body adapts to unaccustomed physical activity, but if you do the same thing indefinitely you lose that stimulus for improvement. So change it up. Even the smallest change can make a positive difference. For example, occasionally try the rowing machine instead of the treadmill, use different resistance training equipment, try a new sport or add a new skill, or even just increase the intensity. Variety and progression are the keys to long-term improvement.

If, in contrast, your 6-week retest shows that you have not made progress, then you should definitely adjust your program. Once again, incorporating some variety may be all it takes to create success. You also may need to increase either the intensity or duration of your activity since it is possible that you are not challenging your body systems enough.

You may be eager to test yourself sooner, but you should understand that you are unlikely to see significant changes before 6 weeks of activity. Naturally, if you have been completely inactive, your performances will improve faster than those of someone who has been active and may be stuck at a plateau. But don't be deceived; your rate of improvement slows as you reach higher levels of fitness, and improving from 20 push-ups to 24 will probably be more difficult than moving from 4 to 12.

MAKING ADJUSTMENTS

At this point, you should have a clear mission, several specific goals, and a plan of action. It is time to begin making changes in your life to increase your personal energy by modifying the fuel you use, the quantity and quality of physical activity you perform, and the recovery and rest you incorporate into your routine. As you get started, remember that even if your plan is well conceived and represents your best intentions, it is likely to need some adjustments as time goes by.

After a period of 2 weeks, step back and evaluate your progress based on your goals, your activity log, and your performance journal. Do you see areas in which you have been too ambitious and need to make your plan more reasonable? Or do you have the opposite case, where you haven't challenged yourself enough?

Consider making small modifications after 2 weeks and at 2-week intervals after that. If you're not sure about a change, tend to stick with your plan for another 2-week period. It may be that you just need a little more time to evaluate your progress.

You might also want to consult with a professional or share your results with another person who can offer an unbiased opinion. Friends who have your best interest at heart may provide helpful sounding boards as you work through this process.

Remember the minimum weekly requirements for physical activity—150 minutes of moderately intense aerobic activity, two strength training sessions with stretching—and consider your weekly schedule. If you cannot do all the activity you originally planned, restart at the minimum level and reset your weekly plan. Perhaps if you are not doing enough, you could simply add an extra activity during the weekend—something recreational and really fun.

If you are just plain short on time, consider increasing the intensity while reducing the duration. Another option is to build in shorter periods of activity during the day, rather than relying on finding an extended period of time. Some people find that simply getting up 30 minutes earlier each day provides the additional time necessary to ensure uninterrupted workout time. You might also try incorporating more physical activity into your workday—for example, by parking farther away from your building to increase your walk to your office or by taking the stairs instead of the elevator.

Frequently Asked Questions

Q: Should I vary the days of the week or time of day for physical activity?

A: This is a common question and one that deserves some reflection. Unquestionably, it is easiest to establish habits and rituals at certain times of the day, and variation often throws us out of kilter. Similarly, picking certain days of the week for activity also works best for most people who have a fairly predictable schedule. If your schedule is predictable, then stick with a regular routine.

It is also true, however, that many of us do not find much predictability during a week or even within certain days. Life simply gets in the way in the form of demands from work, children, social occasions, extemporaneous meetings, traffic, weather, illness, and more. So what to do?

Try to anticipate your schedule and plan your physical activities a week at a time. Schedule them at a time when you predict you'll have the best odds of adhering to the schedule. That's why many people exercise first thing in the morning; it lets them avoid complications. Next, at the end of each day, review your plan for the next day and make schedule adjustments if you know your current activity plans will be foiled. Redo the schedule the night before.

Consider making up missed time in small doses. If you can't squeeze in a 45-minute session, at least go for a 20-minute walk or run. Then add another 15 minutes as soon as you get home that evening. If necessary, choose a different, more convenient activity as a substitute.

Finally, when you miss a scheduled session, make up the time as soon after the missed activity as you can. Don't just throw up your hands and exclaim, "It's not my fault." No, it isn't, but it will be your fault if you do not make up the time.

CREATING HABITS AND RITUALS

We believe that the most effective way to make significant changes in your behavior is to adopt certain rituals and perform them until they become fixed habits. Once you have established a habit, it will be part of your lifestyle and fairly resistant to change (and that is a good thing!).

Most of us believe that we can change our behavior through self-discipline if we just put our mind to it. Sadly, most psychologists agree that only 5 percent of what we do daily is directed by conscious, self-regulated thought (see figure 10.1). The other 95 percent is the result of nonconscious, automatic, or instinctive thought (Bargh and Chartrand 1999). The key to sustained behavior change, then, is to use the limited willpower you do have to establish good habits such as regular physical activity.

If self-discipline is not the key to changing your behavior, then what is? We think it lies in the adoption of certain *rituals of behavior* that you perform daily without much thought or conscious action. You probably have rituals about bedtime, rising in the morning, showering, taking out the trash, driving to familiar places, checking your e-mail, and paying your bills. You don't actually give these things much thought, because you've already committed to them and know that they are important. They are rituals that you've developed.

Think about some of your existing habits, such as brushing your teeth. You don't have to think about doing it or put it on a to-do list; you just automatically do it without any willpower involved. You established this habit a long time ago, and now it would be very difficult for you not to do it. It would, in fact, take a lot of willpower to stop doing it!

This is good news. You don't have to look forward to a life of using self-discipline to adhere to your best prescription for smart nutrition and physical activity. We can promise you that if you adopt a good plan and stick with it for 60 to 90 days, it will become automatic. After that, there will be no question about whether you will eat better or exercise—just decisions about how and when to do so.

If you want to change your patterns of physical activity, diet, sleep, and relaxation, you need to use your 5 percent capacity of self-discipline to make a conscious decision to adopt a new pattern of rituals. Once you have set goals, made a plan, and decided to go for it, you then need only carry it out for a period of 60 to 90 days in order to make it an automatic habit and part of your lifestyle. The longer you continue with the ritual, the more resistant it becomes to change or outside influence.

More to the point, our experience is that once you've established a ritual of physical activity for 60 to 90 days, the chances are excellent that you will continue. Thus, continuing for this period of time should be one of your stated goals at the outset. Go back and look at your goals to determine whether you should add this time line to any of your goals. If 90 days seems too ambitious and daunting, set your sights initially on a smaller amount of time for which you can realistically agree to invest your energy and effort toward your goal.

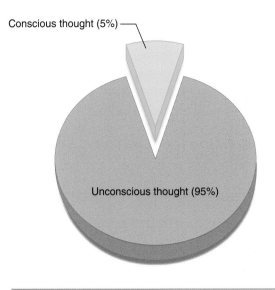

Conscious thought (5%)

Unconscious thought (95%)

Figure 10.1   Conscious and unconscious thought.

If you set a 4-week goal, then at the end of that time you'll be ready to add a few more weeks. Before long, you'll have reached the 60- or 90-day mark, meaning that your habit will be fairly well reinforced and ingrained.

GETTING BACK ON TRACK

At some point, you may fall off the wagon for a few days, or even longer. If so, then, first of all, you are normal. We all have times when we cannot adhere to our intended plans, so rough spots are to be expected to some degree. If you do stumble, think about this: Our clients tell us that the most important thing is not to dwell on the days they missed but to immediately resolve to get back on track the next day.

The key to getting back on track is to remember why you started your physical activity program in the first place. If it was a compelling reason and you focus on it, then it will greatly help you get back on track. For example, if you really enjoy meeting your friends to play tennis twice a week (and you don't forget this fact), this desire will drive you to get back to the tennis courts after a period of inactivity. If you love the energy you get from taking a spinning class, focus on that benefit to help you get yourself back to the gym. You also might find it helpful to recall the feelings of accomplishment you had at the end of a day when you filled out your activity log and journal and were able to recognize good effort toward your goal. Some people find it helpful to post their goals for eating and physical activity in several prominent locations so that they are constantly reminded of them.

It is easy to become discouraged when you fail, but we'd counsel you to have some patience with yourself. Think of the analogy of a young child learning to walk. Her first few tentative efforts at walking are awkward and usually fail, but our response as parents is to celebrate her effort, applaud her spirit of adventure, and encourage her to try again. Imagine the result if we simply said, "You are a failure. Forget it—you'll never be able to walk!" Why not treat yourself and your venture into a healthier lifestyle with that same positive, encouraging, and supportive attitude?

We also think it is critical that you be prepared for periods of time when your activity plan is at risk. For example, if you know you are going to be busy at work for the next 2 weeks, plan for it. For example, commit to performing half of your original physical activity plan during your intense, busy period at work. Even better, resolve to get up 30 minutes earlier for that 2-week period so that following your plan can help you get through the crunch time.

Vacation time can also pose a risk. Before you leave, check out the options for activity wherever you are going; there may be some really fun things to do while you are away! Hiking up a mountain, playing golf, or engaging in a sport (e.g., water or snow sport) that is not available at home can provide the physical activity you need while away. Similarly, plan your dining experiences so that you aren't sucked into eating all types of food in huge portions that are beyond your daily needs or habits at home.

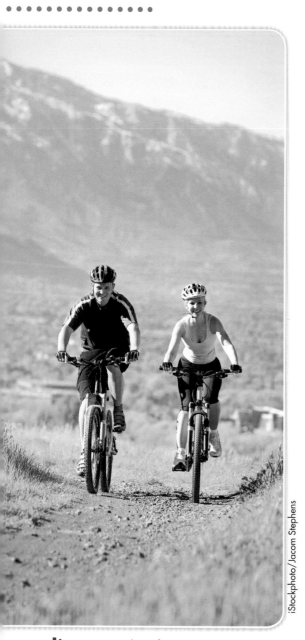

iStockphoto/Jacom Stephens

If you miss a day of activity, get right back on track the next day.

Finally, we hope your physical activity program ultimately becomes one of your many good habits and that, like all habits, it becomes hard *not* to do. Do all that you can to make your physical activity program part of your habitual daily and weekly life and you will ultimately be pulled to do it, no matter the circumstances.

THE MAGIC OF UNINTENDED CONSEQUENCES

One of the great benefits of embarking on a mission to change your behavior is that you will see positive changes and improvements that you didn't plan or anticipate. For example, as you become more active, you may realize that your mood changes are tending toward the positive and that you become more optimistic.

Little things that used to annoy you and cause you to suffer in silence will begin to fade in importance as you refocus your energy on diet, physical activity, and recovery. Chances are excellent that you will also begin to sleep more soundly, due in part to the physical exertion of your activities.

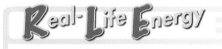

Here's my story. I was overweight at 250 pounds [113 kilograms], I had a high body-fat percentage, and my cholesterol was at 320. My blood glucose was off the charts, and my fitness level was poor. Food and alcohol were my favorite stress relievers. Yo-yo dieting (weight loss and gaining the weight back) was my typical pattern. After enrolling in June in the Corporate Athlete Course at the Human Performance Institute in Orlando, I became very motivated to change my behavior, started eating right, began jogging, and documented my rituals daily.

By autumn, I had fallen back into my old routine of overeating and not exercising. But a few months later, I attended a follow-up refresher course that reignited the flame! My results this time were slow but steady. I really focused on the 40/40/20 peace sign balance of foods and ate low-glycemic snacks regularly. Plus, my colleagues at work encouraged me to sign up to run a half marathon 6 months later. I began to train a couple times a week, increasing my mileage gradually, and completed my first marathon in December. Since then, I've completed two more and also my first triathlon! My statistics now are weight at 205 pounds [93 kg], cholesterol at 150 with no medications, body fat vastly improved, and all blood work normal.

Perhaps even more important, my relationships with my wife and daughter are better than ever, and I have forged many new friendships through my newfound love of running. Professionally, I had the best year of my career in winning Chef of the Year for the Palm Beach Chefs Association, being named Distinguished Visiting Chef at Johnson and Wales University in Miami, and named as Palm Beach Elite in Hospitality Top 100.

—*Jeff Simms, Executive Chef, The Breakers Palm Beach*

Your physical activity will also help you in ways you didn't anticipate or even think to measure. We urged you to measure and evaluate your cardiorespiratory fitness, muscular fitness, flexibility, and body composition, but we know for sure that physical activity offers much more. Here are just a few physical characteristics you may improve through physical activity without even realizing it:

- Static balance
- Dynamic balance
- Agility
- Speed
- Reaction time
- Movement time
- Anticipation
- Core body strength
- Fine motor touch
- Power
- Bone strength
- Bone density

At the same time, you are likely to improve some of your psychosocial characteristics as well:

- Work ethic
- Ability to manage adversity
- Ability to control emotions
- Ability to manage stress
- Problem-solving ability
- Patience with others
- Sporting behavior
- Teamwork
- Independence
- Communication
- Empathy
- Cooperation

In your performance journal, jot down any unintended benefits (whether those just listed or others that you notice) from your new investment of energy and effort into establishing good habits for nutrition, sleep, sport and physical activity, breathing, and recovery.

REWARDING YOURSELF

Positive rewards reinforce your efforts to change. Intrinsic rewards, which engage your inner feelings, are far more powerful than extrinsic rewards over the long term. Your work to stick with your plan, invest effort and energy, stay positive, and complete your activity sessions will produce immediate benefits. Your self-confidence and self-esteem will rise immediately, and you should celebrate this feeling.

That said, we also know that extrinsic rewards can sometimes serve as helpful celebrations of your success, so long as you also have the intrinsic satisfaction. Reward yourself after each week of completing your plan and whenever you achieve either short- or long-term goals.

We suggest that you choose rewards that enhance and reinforce your new commitment rather than undermining it. For example, if you have joined a Pilates class and been a faithful participant, taking a week off is not a good reward.

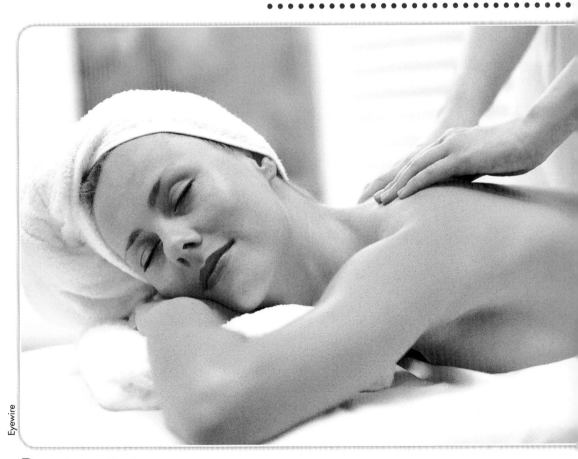

Eyewire

Reward yourself with a great treat.

Likewise, if you've reduced your portions at mealtimes, the reward should not be to pig out for a whole day. Here is a list of rewards that have been effective for many people with whom we have worked.

Massage	New workout clothes
Flowers	Good bottle of wine
Hot tub	New books
New athletic shoes	Biking vacation
Family trip	Dinner with spouse
New bike	New sports equipment
Movie night	Clothing
Manicure or facial	Fresh fruit
Evening with friends	Concert or comedy show
Walk on the beach	Camping in mountains
Karaoke night	Nap
Singing in shower	Music for MP3 player
New gadget	Car wash and detail
Making love	Personal day

You get the idea. You can spice up your life and reward yourself at the same time, and we'll bet that looking forward to the reward helps your energy level immediately.

TIPS for High Energy

- Evaluate and measure your success in developing more personal energy by measuring your progress against your goals.

- Keep a log of your daily performance in which you record your physical activity; also keep a daily journal in which you express your thoughts and feelings along the way.

- At the end of 6 weeks, retest yourself using the same testing procedures used in the beginning and compare your results with your initial scores.

- Invest energy and effort in the rituals and habits you want to cultivate so that they become an automatic part of your new lifestyle.

- Adjust your activities and rituals as necessary, but stick to your commitments of energy and time.

- Reward yourself periodically and celebrate your successes at regular intervals. Invite those close to you to join in these celebrations; their cooperation and support were likely important factors in your achievement.

CHAPTER 11

COMBATING TYPICAL BARRIERS

The endeavor of creating more energy and using it more wisely requires you to overcome some barriers no matter how motivated or passionate you are. That's just life getting in the way. You simply have to expect to encounter obstacles, so it makes sense to actively anticipate them, confront them, and continue to move ahead with your plan for change in your behavior. While we don't want to discourage you before you even begin implementing your plan, we do believe that if you are forewarned of potential barriers, you will be better prepared to address them in a positive way and thus retain the progress you have made. In sport as in life, anticipating problems helps you prepare and sometimes avoid or at least minimize the damage that can be done.

In this chapter, we address typical barriers and suggest strategies for handling them so that they become simply inconveniences rather than causes of failure. We invite you to read this chapter with a hopeful attitude that embraces the notion of being prepared and able to handle any barriers that appear. We also discuss the importance of relaxation and recovery for your mind and body, and we specifically address sleep, which is essential for recovery and for reenergizing your body.

RELAXATION AND RECOVERY

You may recall our explanation (in chapter 1) of the human need for relaxation and recovery. The concept goes hand in hand with the idea that stress is *good* for you and produces growth in every dimension as long as you also build in time for recovery. For example, the only way you can strengthen a muscle is to introduce the stress of using it and in fact overloading it. Within safe limits, the more resistance you provide, the more that muscle is stressed and tested, but the growth and strengthening occur during the rest and recovery phase. Think of your mental, emotional, and spiritual dimensions as having these same qualities—that is, benefiting from stress as long as you provide sufficient time for recovery. In fact, you should embrace the stress you face in any dimension of your being as an opportunity for personal growth.

One barrier that many of us face is a constant diet of stress without adequate time for recovery. It is up to you to anticipate when you will have endured enough stress, whether in your daily life or because of certain extraordinary events, and then plan your recovery time and stick to it.

Recovery time does not necessarily mean withdrawing from all activity. Many times, you just need a change of activity to allow you to recover from the stressor. But be careful about the type of activity you choose, since some apparently relaxing activities produce their own stress. For example, if you remove yourself from stress at work with a few days of vacation but spend it doing frustrating home projects where you feel inadequate and your efforts only produce more anxiety, then you've merely traded one stress for another. A better use of your time away from work is to focus on something that is less challenging, something you thoroughly enjoy that is unlikely to add to your feelings of overwork and fatigue. In a similar vein, we think you should strongly consider physical activity as one of your key strategies for relaxation that allows you to recover from inactivity and the stress of your job.

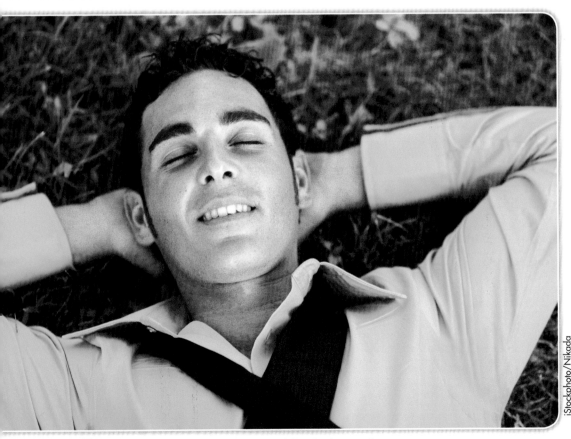

iStockphoto/Nikada

Time for rest and recovery is essential for dealing with stress.

Listening to your favorite music is another surefire way to relax. Research into the effect of music on mood has consistently shown the power of music to enhance relaxation, lift spirits, and energize people and get them moving. If you want to relax, choose a type of music that is calming to you. If you need a pick-me-up, choose music with an upbeat tempo that gets your foot tapping and makes you feel like you just have to move to the rhythm. You can even create a music playlist on your MP3 player that is tailored to fit your activity.

THE POWER OF SLEEP

Nature has blessed us with the amazing power to sleep—a process that provides for rest, relaxation, and growth. But if we try to fool nature by skipping hours of sleep, or if we allow outside factors to interfere with our sleep, we become doomed to enduring lower levels of energy in the days ahead.

Despite individual variation in the optimal number of hours of sleep, certain principles of sleeping are amazingly consistent for most of us. Sleep is a physiological state of the body and mind wherein bodily functions are maintained at a minimal level of energy expenditure. It is a planned period of relative inactivity that allows your brain to process information and your body to grow and repair itself.

According to the (U.S.) National Sleep Foundation, 20 percent of American adults report being so sleepy during the day that it interferes with their daily activities at least a few days a week. What may be worse, 17 percent reported falling asleep while driving within the past year.

In the short term, irregular sleep patterns can lead to lower levels of energy, decreased mental and physical performance quality, and emotional irritability. Lack of sleep may also produce poor decision making and increased risk of accidents, and recent evidence shows that sleep is essential for memory consolidation. Long-term consequences may include increased risk of diabetes, heart disease, obesity, and emotional exhaustion.

Types of Sleep

Sleep can be divided into two major types: REM (or rapid-eye-movement) sleep and NREM (or non-REM, also called *quiet*) sleep. REM sleep is characterized by low-amplitude, high-frequency EEG rhythms, whereas NREM or quiet sleep is characterized by high-amplitude, low-frequency EEG rhythms. EEG rhythms can be simply defined as a measure of electrical activity in the brain.

NREM sleep includes four stages (ranging from light to deep sleep) that we cycle through approximately every 90 minutes. Following each NREM cycle, we then go into REM sleep, the most active stage of sleep and the one in which dreaming often occurs. During REM sleep, the eyes move back and forth beneath the eyelids, and the muscles become immobile. While it is most advantageous to get a full night of sleep, it does appear that the quiet NREM sleep includes a stage of deep sleep that is essential to waking refreshed and energized in the morning.

Your sleep is regulated by a sleep–wake process and by your circadian biological clock (i.e., your 24-hour rhythm that is affected by sunlight). These two systems program our bodies to sleep at night and wake during the day. The sleep–wake process works by determining the amount of sleep you need based on how long you've been awake. Our circadian biological clock regulates hormones such as melatonin, which is secreted during the night and promotes sleep. Generally, children need more sleep than do adults, and older adults need about the same amount of sleep as younger adults, which for most people is 7 to 8 hours of sleep per night.

Frequently Asked Questions

Q: What about taking a nap during the day? Is that a good idea?

A: Chances are that daytime naps are an attempt by your body to catch up on sleep lost during the night. But even if you sleep well at night, you may enjoy the benefits of a short, voluntary nap during the day. Research sponsored by NASA and the Federal Aviation Administration found that strategic 40-minute naps improved subsequent alertness and performance of their personnel. Other research with shift workers and others has shown that even power naps as brief as 20 minutes can improve alertness, psychomotor performance, and mood (Simon 2008).

To get the most benefit from a nap, many people find it best to take it sometime between noon and 4 p.m., which is a good time in the typical sleep–wake cycle. Don't sleep too long—about 20 to 40 minutes works best for most people without keeping them up at night or making them feel groggy—and do give yourself 10 to 15 minutes to wake up before you resume a demanding task. If naps leave you groggy and disoriented or produce nighttime wakefulness, maybe they are not for you (Simon 2008).

According to a Harvard Medical School report, "Doctors used to reassure older people that they needed less sleep than younger ones [in order] to function well, but sleep experts now know that isn't true" (Harvard Health Publications 2008). Older people (like all adults) need 7 to 8 hours of sleep to function at their best; however, falling asleep takes longer for older adults, and they do not get as much deep sleep since they wake repeatedly throughout the night. Consequently, they often supplement their poor sleep with naps during the day.

Improving Your Sleep

You should aim to get 7 to 8 hours of sleep every night with little variation even on weekends. Go to bed and get up at the same time to set your internal clock. Staying up later on weekends and then trying to make up for lost sleep by staying in bed later usually doesn't work; it just confuses your sleep–wake cycle.

Exercising regularly and vigorously promotes deep sleep to repair and grow muscles. You may find that late afternoon or early evening is a good time to exercise, but never do it within 2 hours of bedtime. Exercise stimulates your body, raises your core temperature, and wakes you up. Eventually, as your body cools and lowers your metabolism, you become ready for sleep.

Most sleep experts advise you to eliminate distractions in your bedroom such as bright colors, lights, and television. Keep the room cool, dark, and as quiet as possible. Many people find it a helpful ritual to prepare for bed, then read some relaxing material (not a thriller!) before nodding off. Engaging in intimacy with a partner is also a healthy way to relax and prepare for sleep.

In the evening hours before bedtime, avoid drinks and food with caffeine (e.g., coffee, tea, soda, and chocolate). Alcohol is also problematic since it disrupts sleep stages and acts as a diuretic. In fact, you should limit all fluids in order to minimize nighttime trips to the bathroom. Do not smoke, especially in the 2 hours before bedtime, since nicotine is a stimulant.

What if you have trouble sleeping at night? Here are some remedies to try:

- Take a hot bath before bedtime to draw blood to your skin, cool your body, and lower your metabolism.
- Try deep breathing exercises to relax.
- If you wake up and can't go back to sleep, get up and do something relaxing, such as reading, until you feel sleepy again.

Frequently Asked Questions

Q: Can't I ever have a late night out?

A: Life would be pretty boring if you always kept the same routine and never enjoyed an entertaining night out at a show, movie, concert, or social occasion with friends. The problem is that when you alter your normal sleep routine, you create a sleep debt. The good news, however, is that the debt can be repaid, though not all at once with one long snooze. You'll have to sleep a little longer at night for a few days to get back to normal. A few short daytime naps may also help. So, enjoy your weekend, but pay your debts so that sleep deprivation doesn't become chronic.

- Be sure to get adequate exercise during the day to tire your body naturally.
- Eat a smaller meal at night to allow your internal processes to shut down as well.

Finally, falling asleep while watching television and then waking up to go to bed is fairly likely to disturb your natural sleep cycle. It's better to just go to bed when you've reached your limit.

NUTRITION CHALLENGES

Every day, we face challenges in the food choices we have to make—what to eat, when to eat it, and how much to eat. Here are several typical challenges:

- Large portions served at home or in restaurants
- Foods high in unhealthy content such as sugar and trans fat
- Irregular meals due to work schedule or family responsibilities
- Lack of healthy snack food (and presence of junk food snacks)

A rereading of chapter 3 (Adding High-Octane Fuel), will help you recall the principles of eating properly to produce energy for your body. Once you understand and accept these principles, you are on your way to overcoming the challenges. We encourage you, however, to continue to learn and explore healthy options for your daily diet by reading, listening to experts, and sharing ideas with interested friends.

We strongly urge that you to take charge of your own nutrition rather than leaving yourself at the whim of whoever happens to prepare your food, whether at home or in a restaurant. You should probably shop for your own snacks; see what the options are and choose healthy snacks that appeal to you. You may also find that doing some shopping around in the grocery store gives you ideas for healthier foods, enlarges your number of choices, and helps you plan better menus even if you are not doing the meal preparation yourself.

If meal preparation at home is done by someone else, you simply have to enlist his or her support in making the dietary adjustments you want to make. Ask, beg, or bribe—but get his or her agreement to help you. In fact, the person may need to change some of his or her own behavior, perhaps choosing different foods, preparing smaller portions, and opting for better snack choices.

When you go to a restaurant, know what you want to order and how it should be prepared. Ask for special consideration from the chef and eliminate the extra calories contained in bread or appetizers unless they fit into your five allowable handfuls. Share a meal with someone else in order to reduce your portion, or ask for a carryout container as soon as your meal is delivered and eat only half of the portion at the restaurant.

Be especially careful about alcohol when dining out. Having a drink before dinner, wine with the meal, and an after-dinner drink clearly add unneeded calories. Remember that just one glass of wine at dinner should substitute for a handful of grains if you want to keep your portions under control.

Although social rituals in some circles include several alcoholic drinks before, during, and after meals, we urge you to sip nonalcoholic drinks instead. Water or some variation of it is clearly the best option.

WORK AND LIFE COMMITMENTS

At certain times in our lives, commitments at work or personal life simply take extraordinary amounts of time and energy. In such situations, our natural tendency is to cut back on exercise routines, sleep less, and resort to comfort foods to get us through tough times, but these behaviors only exacerbate the extraordinary demands on our energy, thus forcing our bodies to work even harder in order to compensate.

When responsibilities at work or home become extraordinary, this is the time to exert the limited self-discipline we have and maintain the positive rituals we have put in place. If you've done a good job of establishing healthy rituals, they will be reasonably resistant to change and will allow you to cope with almost any emergency.

Suppose, for instance, that you have reached a critical time at work where your responsibilities unexpectedly spiral into a crisis. How should you respond? Choose an answer from the following options.

   a. Fully dedicate yourself to the crisis, immerse yourself in finding solutions, and ignore your personal needs until the crisis has passed.
   b. Analyze the crisis and develop an action plan with successive steps leading to a potential solution.
   c. Panic! Worry about the situation, think about it constantly, and expect things to get worse before they get better!
   d. Step back, evaluate the severity of the crisis, plan for action, and take care of your personal energy and health while you cope with the situation.

Depending on which choices you make, the short- and long-term effects of any crisis are likely to be magnified if you ignore your personal energy and health needs. We recommend that you follow the strategy described in option d.

Remember that your body needs the fuel from healthy food, water, and exercise in order to function optimally in normal times; when you face pressure and stress, those needs don't change. The fact is that you think more clearly, work more efficiently, and sleep better if you monitor your eating, exercise, and recovery time even during a work crisis. Make time for your normal rituals and stick to them so that your body and mind can operate efficiently and effectively.

Times of personal crisis call for a similar response. We are all challenged at some point in life by traumatic events such as the diagnosis of a severe health problem in a loved one, a death in the family, divorce, loss of a job, surviving a hurricane or tornado, or a financial setback. Athletes and (even more so) members of the military engage in intense training so that they can meet the large and critical demands of their jobs. The greater the demands, the better the training needs to be. Don't skimp on your own training (i.e., exercise, nutrition, rest, and sleep) when times get tough. It is precisely during these times of extreme stress that you must rely on your personal rituals and training to provide structure to help you weather the storm. Maintaining your fitness and your high energy level surely helps you through life's greatest challenges.

We recommend that you stick to your time-tested routines as much as possible in order to equip yourself with the physical, mental, emotional, and spiritual energy to confront the crisis. Keep in mind that your work to develop healthy rituals was not done just for normal times but also to serve you well in an emergency. If your habits of healthy living have been well established over time, they will be resistant to change from any source and will provide the structure you can use to handle any crisis.

Frequently Asked Questions

Q: What if I blow my energy program during an extreme family or work emergency?

A: Let's face it—it does happen. But there is nothing to be gained by self-flagellation over past actions. Accept the fact that some situations challenge even our strongest commitments and rituals. Now it's time to move on.

Begin implementing your renewed commitment to your rituals for better health and energy as soon as possible. Regard the momentary lapse as just that and get back on track—the sooner you return to your plan, the better. The fact that you already have a plan in place and know what actions to take gives you a head start on resuming your program.

HEALTH ISSUES

You may be moving along nicely in your new program of rituals for health and fitness, then suddenly find yourself facing illness or injury. Both of these outside factors can have an immediate and prolonged effect on your diet and exercise plans and even cause you to lose all the momentum you've built toward achieving a higher energy level.

Your initial reaction to either an injury or an illness is likely to be the notion that you need rest, and that may be true. Performing at a high level is challenging even when you are healthy. But rest may not be the best prescription in every case.

If your illness manifests itself from your neck up in the form of a head cold, there's no harm in continuing to exercise; in fact, you may well feel better if you get moving and stimulate your bodily systems, though you might need to adjust the intensity or duration of activity sessions while you are sick. If, on the other hand, you are feeling an illness somewhere in the body from the neck down, it's probably wise to curtail your physical activity until you feel better, then limit the intensity or duration of your sessions as you build up to normal capacity.

Injuries are tricky, and you want to be sure that you don't exacerbate an injury and turn it into a chronic problem. You may need to seek advice from a medical professional who can evaluate the severity of your injury and prescribe treatment. If you don't see quick significant improvement in an injury, we recommend that you get medical advice soon in order to prevent complications or a lingering or chronic problem.

Generally, you should follow the PRICE principle—Prevention, Rest, Ice, Compression, and Elevation—for most injuries. Avoid using heat until at least 48 hours have passed, since heat only adds to any swelling that may occur.

In the case of many injuries, aggressive treatment by a sports medicine professional can minimize the negative effect and prevent a long-term problem. In addition, strengthening the surrounding muscles and improving flexibility can help you recover faster and reduce the odds of further injury. If you simply rest an injury too long, you'll lose strength and flexibility, thus making reinjury more likely.

Our best advice is to visit your medical provider and follow the recommended treatment so that you can resume your physical activity as soon as possible. It will be a poor choice if you decide to simply ignore an injury and press on with your activity. This approach may lead to further damage and prolong the injury. Equally unwise is to simply rest without treatment or rehabilitation; if you do this, you're simply sliding backward, and your recovery time will be extended.

TRAVEL

For those who travel to do business, perhaps nothing is more daunting than trying to maintain a healthy lifestyle when living on the road. The traveling itself can drain our energy and leave us feeling fatigued and more eager to nap than exercise. If you have to cross time zones, jet lag can leave you feeling disoriented, and you may find that the last thing you want to think about is your fitness program. Fortunately, you can take certain steps to counter these potential pitfalls of travel, renew your personal energy, and be physically active wherever you land.

Physical Effects of Travel

First, let's look at the cause of travel fatigue. As discussed earlier in this book, your blood transports glucose and oxygen to your body's cells, where energy is generated. Thus, anything that compromises your blood's ability to deliver glucose and oxygen limits your ability to generate energy, and herein lies the problem: The circulation of your blood is severely affected by travel, especially by sitting in one position on an airplane for hours at a time.

The largest muscle in your body, in your buttocks, is suppressed by sitting, thus minimizing blood flow through your buttocks to your legs and feet and back up to your heart, lungs, and brain. This lack of proper circulation may cause your muscles to tingle, become numb, feel asleep, or even become painful.

Prolonged sitting or inactivity also causes a decrease in body metabolism. Your metabolism is simply the rate at which you generate energy; it increases when you move, but in order to conserve energy it decreases when you are inactive. The result of a lowered metabolism is a feeling of fatigue and lethargy.

The solution to both impaired circulation and decreased metabolism is to *move!* Your body is meant to move, and movement enhances your circulation and metabolism at the same time. Anytime you find yourself inactive for a long time while traveling, get up and find a way to move in order to increase your energy. Here are some tips for doing so through stretching, small muscle movements, and large muscle movements.

- Stretching releases muscle tension, improves blood flow, and decreases muscle discomfort. Try reaching with both arms above your head, or straight out in front of you; you might also try pulling one knee at a time to your chest. For each stretch, hold the position for 15 to 30 seconds and breathe normally.

- Small muscle movements also increase blood flow, elevate your metabolism, and help you relax. Two moves you can do while sitting are (1) rolling your shoulders forward and backward and (2) doing small arm circles.

- Large movements have the greatest effect on your systems, and they require that you get up from a sitting position and move around. On an airplane, you can use the aisle or the area in the back of the plane to walk, stretch, touch your toes, reach for the sky, or perform large arm circles. Gently twist and turn your body; stretch each muscle group in your arms, legs, and torso.

Whether you are riding on an airplane or train, traveling by automobile, or sitting at your desk for long periods, we suggest that you do the following:

- Perform some stretching every 30 to 45 minutes.
- Perform large muscle movements every 90 to 120 minutes.
- Get up and move by walking at least every 2 hours.

Handling Jet Lag

Your body has established certain rhythms and routines for sleep, rest, and mealtime, and it is sensitive to light and darkness. These routines are shattered when you travel across time zones; it confuses your body and mind. A trip halfway around the world will cause you to adjust by about 12 hours, making night seem like day and vice versa. Such trips take a toll on your energy and may also cause headaches, stomach pain, difficulty in concentrating, dizziness, and disruption of both duration and quality of sleep. It usually takes about 1 day to adjust for each time zone you cross.

Here are our recommendations for minimizing problems with jet lag:

- *If possible, keep to your home schedule.* On short trips involving just one or two time zones, schedule appointments for times when you would be alert at home and ignore the time change if you will be gone for just a day or two.
- *If crossing more than two time zones, switch to the new time zone before your trip.* Move your sleep and your mealtimes before you depart in order to give your body a chance to gradually adjust. If possible, arrive at your destination a day early to allow yourself time to adjust before you have to perform professionally.
- *Resist the temptation to sleep once you arrive.* Switch immediately to local time and keep yourself active until bedtime. Spend time outdoors to let daylight reset your internal clock.
- *Use sunlight to reset your internal rhythms.* If you need to wake earlier (after flying from west to east), get out in the early morning sun. If you need to wake later (after flying from east to west), expose yourself to late afternoon sun.
- *Drink plenty of fluids during travel, but not caffeine or alcohol.* Both worsen the symptoms of jet lag and can disturb sleep patterns.
- *Consider melatonin.* The level of melatonin in your body rises naturally at night in order to promote sleep and decreases during the day to keep you awake. On long trips, melatonin supplements (available from any drugstore) may help you shift your circadian rhythm more easily.
- *Use exercise to your advantage.* Exercising stimulates your metabolism, releases hormones that promote alertness, and enhances the quality of sleep. If nothing else, once you arrive at your destination, take a vigorous walk or run at least 3 hours before bedtime.

Maintaining Physical Activity Away From Home

Many business travelers tell us that once they've established a routine for regular physical activity at home, their downfall occurs when they travel. Schedules are tight, facilities are unfamiliar, and exercise buddies are in short supply. But don't wimp out now. You've invested too much energy into increasing your regular physical activity to let it slip away.

Expect to meet challenges in your efforts to continue physical activity while traveling, and plan accordingly to ensure success. Be creative and committed to keeping your energy level high throughout your trip. Here are some suggestions:

- *Exercise before you leave home* so that you have earned some recovery time. Incorporate time for physical activity into your preparation before your trip.

- *Check out hotel facilities before you leave home.* Pick hotels that cater to business travelers by providing gyms, running or walking paths, swimming pools, or tennis courts. Even if exercise facilities are not offered on site, most hotels can recommend nearby facilities.

- *Pack workout shoes and clothing and, if appropriate for you, a swimsuit.* Be prepared for a variety of options depending on available facilities, time, and your mood.

- *Pack your tunes.* Bring your favorite upbeat music and earphones for use during your physical activity. You'll look forward to changing your mood through music and reenergizing yourself by combining movement with music.

- *Pack a resistance band.* These elastic bands are light, easy to pack, and useful for getting a full-body strength workout right in your hotel room.

- *Bring along a workout video.* Many good workout videos are available to stimulate you while you move, even in a hotel room. You can store a video on your laptop or rent a video player at your hotel. Choose from Pilates, yoga, and aerobics workouts that are available online or at big-box stores for less than US$20.

- *Pack a portable fitness program.* PowerHouse Hit the Deck includes an interval timer and 35 cards, each showing a specific exercise that needs no special equipment. It's available from www.powerhousehit thedeck.com.

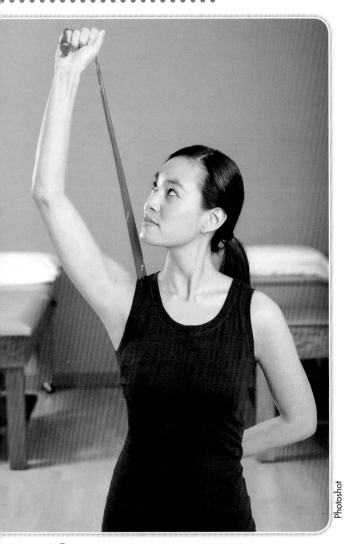

Photoshot

A resistance band can provide a great strength training workout anywhere you travel.

Once you are on-site, check out the available options for physical activity and plan your time. If you are dealing with time changes, you'll find natural times when you could squeeze in a workout, perhaps early in the morning or during the late afternoon. Even if you have only 10 to 20 minutes for physical activity, making good use of this time can make a difference in your energy level and help you maintain your fitness level. Consider shaving some minutes off of time spent in the hotel bar or otherwise socializing in order to get your physical activity done.

As we see it, here are the options for physical activity on the road. All of these venues can work effectively, and you might enjoy the variety of trying different ones.

- *Outdoors.* You can walk, jog, or run. Make it a sightseeing venture and enjoy the new scenery. Consider walking to appointments, meetings, or meals.
- *Hotel or nearby gym or other facility.* Hotel gyms often provide both cardiorespiratory and strength training equipment. For fun, try equipment that is different from what you use in your routine back home. Swimming can be both relaxing and vigorous whether done indoors or outside.
- *Hotel stairs.* Hotels always have stairs, and you can use them for activity. Try running or walking a few flights for a challenging workout, but don't forget to stretch before and after.
- *Your room.* Use your own body weight in your hotel room for stretching and strength training. Even in limited space, you can make good use of push-ups, squats, lunges, and crunches. Consider using PowerHouse Hit the Deck (mentioned on page 200) in your room or outdoors for a crisp 20- to 30-minute workout that will get your heart pumping.

After a packed day of doing business, you can rejuvenate yourself through stretching and deep breathing. Consider treating yourself to a warm bath, whirlpool, or massage as a reward for being physically active on the road.

INTERPERSONAL BARRIERS

We live and work with all kinds of people. Some of them seem to sap our personal energy and, even more disappointing, may prevent us from replenishing our supply. Take stock of the relationships in your life that seem to interfere with your commitment to better nutrition and more physical activity and develop a strategy to enlist the support of those around you.

You may be shocked to learn that some people around you may try to sabotage your healthy lifestyle changes just because they resist change of any kind. Their lack of support may be conscious or unconscious, but either way it can derail your good intentions. Lack of support from others may also be rooted in their own feelings of inadequacy if they know that they too should be engaging in more physical activity. They may even feel that you are implicitly criticizing their behavior or sending a message that there is trouble in your relationship. In any case, the question is this: What can you do to gain their support?

The answer starts with being forthcoming about your commitment to developing healthier habits. People who care about you will usually be supportive unless your plan interferes with their convenience. If your time for physical activity replaces family time, then you need to point out the benefits to everyone of your having more energy to engage with them after you are active. Better yet, invite them to join you if appropriate.

Co-workers may be less understanding and may even resent the time you devote to your personal health. Your supervisor may demand your time unreasonably, especially if he or she feels pressure from his or her supervisors. You may have to negotiate smartly when work demands are heavy and you realize that your performance is affected by fatigue and lack of energy. Tactfully point out to work colleagues that you'll be more productive if you're physically active and therefore healthier, happier, and better able to perform on the job.

Social friends and extended family simply may not be as interested in or aware of your commitment to nutrition and physical activity. To avoid awkward situations and confrontations, it's best to make plans that factor in your needs and lifestyle changes. Inquire ahead of time about social occasions, choice of restaurants, and plans for meals and try to anticipate trouble spots.

Frequently Asked Questions

Q: What happens if I am invited to a special occasion, such as a wedding, birthday, or just a regular social gathering?

A: Most people celebrate special occasions with food—often large quantities of food. Alcohol may be added to the equation, and the whole event can last forever. For those of us who are trying to be conscious of our nutrition habits, these are times that try our souls.

Our advice is to know what to expect and to plan your strategy. Eat a snack beforehand so that you are not hungry and are not tempted to drink alcohol on an empty stomach. Plan your alcohol consumption ahead of time and keep a careful eye on your glass lest it get magically refilled without your noticing.

Sip diet tonic water or a diet soft drink during cocktail hour and limit your hors d'oeuvres to one or two items. Once the food is served, limit your portion size, but try as many different dishes as you like with small servings. Even unhealthy or rich foods can be tolerated if portions are tiny.

Skip the dessert and after-dinner drinks unless you sip and share with your spouse. Excuse yourself to the rest room at least once if necessary to break away from the food orgy and move around during the event.

If you can convince others to adjust plans a bit, you'll be happier and they won't be disappointed. If you find yourself in a situation you can't control, such as a family wedding, it may be up to you to adjust your habits for one day and make the best of it.

BOREDOM AND BURNOUT

People who monitor fitness programs at health and fitness clubs regularly report that more than half of their clients quit the program within the first year. The fact is that adopting a healthy lifestyle through diet and physical activity takes time—time to plan a beginning and time to solidify habits and routines. But it doesn't stop there. You have to constantly support and nourish your activity program throughout your life in order to fully integrate it into your lifestyle.

Think about planting a new shrub or bush in your yard. You need to carefully choose the location, prepare the soil, fertilize it, and add a generous amount of water at the first planting. During the succeeding weeks, you check on the plant's growth and water it as needed. Even after your new planting has firmly established roots and seems to be growing healthily, you can't just ignore it. You still need to provide periodic feedings to help the plant maintain its health, water it during dry spells, and trim it periodically to ensure long-term survival as a healthy plant. Your program for physical activity demands no less.

After performing a routine for some weeks, the early excitement may wear off, and you may begin to feel bored. Periodic retesting for progress helps motivate you to maintain or step up the intensity of your training. In addition, as suggested in earlier chapters, celebrations or rewards can provide extrinsic motivation, but even those lose their effectiveness over time.

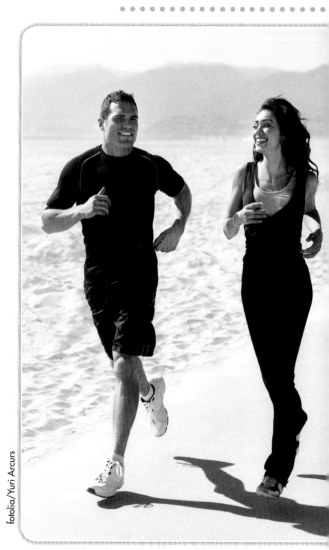

fotolia/Yuri Arcurs

Physical activity with a partner helps you to avoid boredom and burnout.

If you feel bored with your program, the key is to change it up before the problem leads to slacking off. Vary your sites for workouts, the equipment you use, and your methods of activity. Seek out new friends or exercise partners who spark your interest and give you positive reinforcement. Set new goals every few weeks and dedicate yourself to achieving them. Expect to be bored eventually, but plan for it and strategize so that your boredom is only a momentary blip on your screen.

Invest some time in learning a new physical activity that captures your imagination. Adding new skills boosts your confidence, provides variety, and exposes you to a whole new culture of activity converts. Add some competition so that you have specific events to focus on, such as an Ironman, a 10K run, a marathon, the state senior games, or an age-defined competition in any sport. Similarly, planning to participate in a charity walk or local fun run, or even playing in a flag football tournament at your local recreation center, can add a competitive and fun element to your activity program.

You might also consider investing in new technology or sports equipment that enhances your workouts and increases your enthusiasm. A new golf club, tennis racket, pair of in-line skates, bicycle, or scuba gear can boost your excitement and improve performance.

The curse of burnout is more difficult to deal with. Burnout may have a physical, psychological, or emotional cause, but regardless of the cause it involves a devastating feeling of frustration. Most of us identify burnout as a hazard facing high-performance elite athletes who simply become unable to meet the excessive demands of training or competing at an elite level. However, all physically active people are at risk for burnout.

Burnout victims often feel exhausted and lose their energy and their interest in physical activity. They begin to feel low self-esteem and a sense of failure, and they may become depressed. Classic causes of burnout include intense stress, physical fatigue, boredom, muscle soreness, injury, and lack of proper rest and sleep. Clearly, our advice to incorporate recovery time into your schedule deserves mention here as a strategy for avoiding the causes of burnout.

Our advice for avoiding burnout is to plan your physical activity in cycles of relatively high-intensity activity followed by rest and then a return to activity at a moderate level. Using the natural rhythms of your body as a guide, alternate heavy and light workout days and periodically intensify your activity in preparation for an event or competition of some type. After peaking for competition, take a few days off and substitute light activity and stretching for maintenance. Cross-train by using a totally different sport activity that still keeps you moving. Tennis players might head to the golf course, runners might jump in the pool, and dancers might take a yoga class to vary their routines.

Both boredom and burnout can be nipped early if you are conscious of their presence and plan strategies for coping with them. If you go more than a few days without feeling energized by physical activity, heed the warning and analyze your feelings. Once you've identified your feelings and the possible causes, adjust your physical activity plan to head off trouble.

TIPS for High Energy

- Consciously incorporate time for rest and recovery into your routines.
- Aim for adequate hours of sleep of good quality and stick to a routine as much as possible.
- Plan for challenges to your nutrition plan (from social and holiday celebrations as well as dining out) by adopting specific strategies to avoid overeating or excessive drinking.
- Be smart about travel by incorporating physical activity into your trip agenda.
- Take illness and injury seriously and seek expert medical help where appropriate to prevent long-term interference with your physical activity plan.
- Accept the fact that family and friends may not be uniformly supportive of your plan for enhanced energy and learn to actively enlist their cooperation.
- Prepare for possible boredom or burnout in your physical activity and develop strategies to minimize the effect.

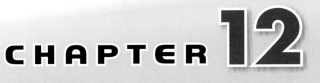

CHAPTER 12

PLANNING FOR THE FUTURE

Without a clear plan for the future, it is quite possible that you will begin implementing your personal plan to enhance your energy but after a few weeks or months hit a plateau or even begin to slide backward into old habits. In order to prevent that from happening, now is the time to reinforce your primary mission, which should be about increasing your personal energy and managing it more effectively.

In this chapter, we help you review the key concepts of personal energy management and the principles for successful change. With these thoughts in mind, you'll have a strong foundation on which to develop a long-term plan that increases your odds of succeeding during the months and years ahead.

Specifically, this chapter helps you strengthen your intrinsic motivation to change your behavior and nurture that motivation for the long term in spite of obstacles that arise. We also introduce you here to the value and purpose of becoming your own coach by building your personal understanding and skills to enhance and manage your personal energy. Finally, we help you learn how to build an effective support team to encourage, support, and push you through the months to come.

REVIEWING KEY CONCEPTS

You started this journey at the beginning of this book by reading and thinking about your personal energy crisis. It is virtually certain that in today's world you often feel a lack of energy but are uncertain of what to do about it. Our recommendations throughout this book are geared toward helping you accomplish the mission of creating more personal energy and managing it better. The strategies for generating more energy are rooted in the sciences of nutrition and exercise physiology. As a result, most of the advice in this book has addressed three topics: choosing what to eat and drink, adopting a regular plan for physical activity, and establishing time for rest and recovery.

At the outset, we made it clear that although you may feel pressed for time, *time is really not the issue.* You have only 24 hours a day to work with, and while you might do better at managing your time by setting priorities and sequencing tasks, you'll still have only 24 hours.

Generating More Physical Energy

Our physical selves allow us to generate energy from the *nutrients* we ingest, from the quality and quantity of *recovery* times we build into our schedules, and from *physical activity.* Let's review each of these major factors briefly.

Nutrition   You need to take in oxygen, water, and glucose in order to provide the physical energy needed for living. We've offered hints for using each of these raw materials most efficiently by describing the need, the best strategies for intake, and the effect on your energy.

In short, you need to learn to regulate your nutrition habits especially when you feel pressure. Virtually all of us need to take in more water than we do on a consistent basis; we also need to increase our intake when we are physically active. Finally, we need to regulate our intake and our use of glucose by eating light and often. You can keep your glucose at a consistent level throughout the day by eating three regular meals of five handfuls each, as well as two between-meals snacks.

Physical Activity   We've built our whole strategic framework for physical activity around the concept of having fun. We believe that physical movement is critical to generating physical energy and achieving fitness, but if it is perceived as a chore or as work you're much more likely to avoid it. Our strategy is to carefully choose physical activities that are fun, whatever that means to you. We've identified (in

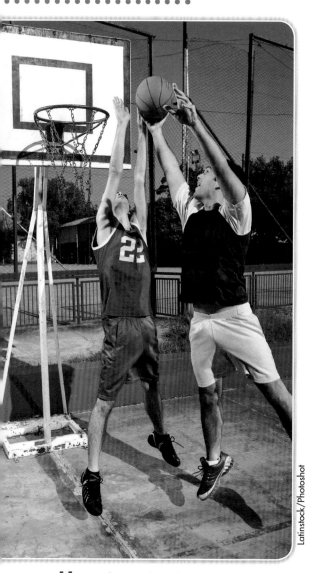

Having fun is a key element to getting yourself motivated.

Latinstock/Photoshot

chapter 6) the types of fun that might attract you, and we've provided an exhaustive list of possible physical activities for you to choose from.

To assess your present level of physical fitness, we've prescribed simple but effective physical tests that you can self-administer and use to compare your results with national standards. Once you've established your personal baseline, you need to plan for regular physical activity that will improve your cardiorespiratory fitness, muscular strength and endurance, flexibility, and body composition.

Recovery   You need to incorporate regular cycles of recovery time to offset the expenditure of energy each day. The quality and quantity of sleep is the basis for renewal, and its importance cannot be ignored. The healthiest attitude accepts stress as a helpful and necessary part of everyday life that allows us to accomplish goals. But unless you also take time for recovery from daily stress, your body will eventually succumb to stress. Recovery time may be well spent in physical activity, since activity can be a powerful stress reducer, provided that you enjoy the activity.

Using Energy More Effectively

Let's return briefly to the concept of full engagement that was explained in chapter 1. We defined full engagement as an acquired ability to invest your full and best energy right here, right now. This is an *acquired* skill—something you can learn.

We highlighted the importance of the present, which is the only time we can invest energy. It is not possible to invest energy in the past, as that time has already gone (though your history does, of course, indicate where you have previously invested energy). The future holds promise only if you invest energy in the present to plan for the future. While it is not helpful to worry or be anxious about the future, smart planning now can set you on a good path for meeting future energy demands.

Thus the question is this: What should I invest my energy in at the present time?

Our response is that your full and best energy should be expended toward establishing habits that maximize your production of personal energy and allow you to use it efficiently. Invest in rituals (which are conscious behaviors requiring willpower and self-discipline) such as eating breakfast, eating snacks between meals, getting regular physical exercise, and enabling restful sleep. After a time, these rituals will become established or embedded habits that are automatic and require no conscious behavior.

It is also crucial to incorporate time for recovery after stress in order to allow your body and mind time to grow and prepare for the next stressful activity. If you constantly drain energy resources without replenishing the supplies, eventually your body and mind will rebel and insist on recovery time that is out of your control.

MOTIVATING YOURSELF

Lack of strong, pervasive intrinsic motivation usually results in a failure to adopt new habits of healthier living (e.g., better nutrition choices, regular physical activity, and planned recovery time). While we do acknowledge the temporary benefits of extrinsic rewards for achievement of new habits, the longer-lasting effect of intrinsic motivation is far superior over time (for in-depth treatment of motivation, reread chapter 4).

Reconnect your motivation to the purpose that you see for your life. Reflect on your sense of why you are here on Earth and what you identify as your mission in life. If your mission is to be the best possible mother to your children, for example, then make that the foundation of your motivation to live a healthier lifestyle. You will benefit directly and immediately as a parent, and you will become a powerful role model for your children as they grow and mature.

In chapter 10, we urged you to create and write your *personal mission for change*. It may be something like this: "To create more personal energy so that I am more productive at work and more engaged with my family during non-working hours." Review your personal mission now, then think about strategies you could adopt to ensure that you keep your mission at the forefront during the months ahead. Would it be helpful to post it in prominent places? Insert it in your daily calendar to force you to review it daily? Perhaps use it as your screensaver? Put it on the dashboard of your car?

Next, review the more specific goals you've set. These goals should include a timeline for achievement and imply an urgency to accomplish them. Here is a sample goal: "Each Sunday, I will plan and schedule my physical activity for the coming week, thus giving it the priority it deserves in my life."

Your plan for the future should be constructed on the solid, realistic, but hopeful foundation of your personal mission for change and the specific goals you have set. Taking this approach will help you keep moving forward on the path you've chosen for the future. Keep in mind that your strongest intrinsic motivation to persevere comes from examining and prioritizing your personal values and from the resulting goals you set.

Even as you reflect upon your life mission and long-term goals, keep sight of the significance of the journey you have embarked upon. Learn to treasure the value of the journey itself and be thankful for the daily opportunities it presents. Once again, if you stay present-centered you will be able to expend your personal energy most effectively.

BECOMING YOUR OWN COACH

You may feel woefully inadequate to the task of becoming your own coach, but you have more knowledge of yourself and a better understanding of your personal challenges than anyone else does. Coaches do not necessarily have all the answers, but they do have the knowledge and skill to clearly identify chal-

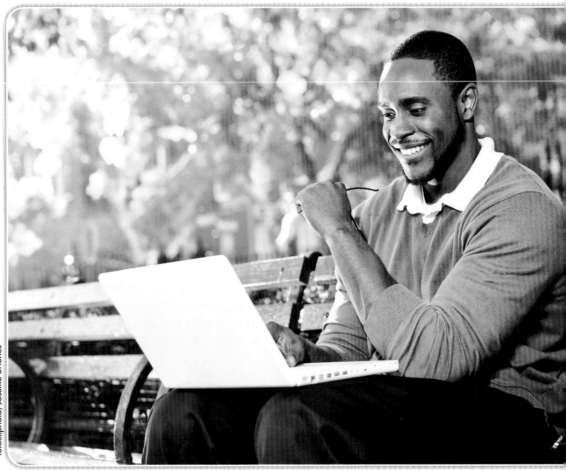

You can become your own coach by continuing to learn and plan your strategy for more energy.

lenges and help construct a game plan to address each challenge. We are not suggesting that you forgo consultation with experts in related fields, but that only you can take their suggestions and integrate them into a plan that works for you. A helpful analogy might be to think of yourself as a head football coach who relies on advice and counsel from the team's athletic trainer, physician, offensive coach, defensive coach, and special teams coach in constructing an overall game plan each week. As the head coach for your own plan, you have the final responsibility to make decisions that increase your chances of success.

What you might be lacking in this analogy is a complete and thorough understanding of the principles of energy management and of various strategies for developing better rituals and habits. Thus we urge you to reread sections of this book periodically to refresh your memory and perhaps deepen your understanding. You might also consider enrolling in the Corporate Athlete Course offered by the Human Performance Institute for an intense 2 1/2 days of training in the concepts and application of personal energy management.

We also suggest that you continue to read and learn about nutrition, physical activity, recovery, and related topics. As you encounter new information, analyze it carefully and compare it with your current understanding and experience to discern whether this new information might help or hinder your progress toward your personal goals. We urge you to give more weight to information that is supported by sound research replicated by various groups over time and research that has been endorsed by such reputable organizations as a government agency (e.g., the Centers for Disease Control and Prevention) or national professional organizations (e.g., the American College of Sports Medicine). Be skeptical of claims from a lone practitioner who is promoting a method or product for personal financial gain that is not grounded in responsible scientific research.

It is also helpful to have a circle of trusted advisors who are experienced and well educated in sport and the exercise sciences. These advisors might include people who specialize in exercise physiology, sports medicine, sport psychology, nutrition, physical training and fitness, and physical therapy. When you encounter new ideas, strategies, or practices, ask your advisors for their guidance and recommendations based on their expertise.

You can use the following frequently asked questions, complete with references to previous chapters, to highlight information you need to learn in order to serve effectively as your own coach.

Question: How do I find more hours in the day to exercise?

Answer: You will never be able to add hours to your day, but you can certainly set priorities and become more efficient during the hours you do have. Review the portion of chapter 8 that discusses dividing your activity times into small segments that, taken together, total up to the amount of time each day that you should be physically active.

Question: How will I know if I am making improvements in my physical fitness?

Answer: Review the discussion in chapter 5 about methods for testing your levels of fitness. We suggest that you retest yourself at 6-week intervals to allow yourself sufficient time to make fitness gains. When you do the retests, make certain that the circumstances and testing activities are replicated exactly from the initial test. This means testing in the same environment, at the same time of day, and after eating a similar meal.

Question: My physical activities are becoming boring, and I think I need a change to stay motivated. What other activities should I consider?

Answer: Go back to chapter 6 and consider the environment and the types of physical activity that appeal to you. Pick several and experiment with them to see which ones seem to be a good fit. Keep in mind that it may take some time to become comfortable with and skillful in performing the new activity, so don't write off a choice prematurely.

Question: I constantly feel that other people, work demands, and life in general are getting in the way of my new program for physical activity. How can I work around these strong outside influences?

Answer: Review chapter 11, which presents the typical barriers and suggests strategies for working through or around them. Be creative in approaching perceived barriers and developing alternative solutions.

Question: Even though I am now physically active, my stress level is still extremely high. What can I do to reduce the stress I feel?

Answer: Review chapter 4 to be sure that you understand the concept that stress can be a positive factor only if it is combined with time for recovery. Check your daily schedule to ensure that you are incorporating sufficient recovery and rest time. Also evaluate whether it is possible that your current physical activity adds to your stress rather than reducing it. For example, if you really don't enjoy the activity you are doing, it can be a stressor. Or if your golf scores are consistently rising, perhaps you need to either take a break from golf or arrange for lessons in hopes of improving your performance.

Question: Where can I get more extensive information about nutrition that is based on scientific research rather than on a commercial product someone is trying to sell me?

Answer: Order a copy of *Nancy Clark's Sports Nutrition Guidebook, Fourth Edition* (2008, Human Kinetics, Champaign, IL). You'll find lots of relevant information for physically active people.

Question: I need some variety in the type of strength training exercises I do. Where can I get more information about alternative workout routines?

Answer: Try using various types of strength training equipment, including machines, free weights, resistance bands, medicine balls, Swiss or exercise balls, and your own body weight. Consider taking up Pilates or yoga in a group workout once a week or buy a video and follow the workout routine. Use a training circuit but change the exercises you do during each workout (while still making sure to work each muscle group). You might also consult with a certified fitness professional, explain your goals and current program, and ask for some alternatives.

Question: Every time I get started on a good path, something else in life comes up to ruin it and I have to start all over again. How can I avoid these constant crises and deal with them when they do occur?

Answer: Go back to the discussion in chapter 11 about typical barriers and strategies for handling periods when you feel compelled to suspend your program for activity.

To become a truly effective personal coach, you need to keep learning and growing in your knowledge and understanding of the principles, strategies, and techniques for better energy management. Now that you know what is involved and have implemented your program, it will become apparent where you have gaps in knowledge or understanding. Continue to read materials from the library or search the World Wide Web for relevant articles. If you have already completed the Corporate Athlete Course, consider taking a refresher course at the Human Performance Institute.

While you are continuing on your personal program, consider learning new sports skills or trying new physical activities that could add variety to your program. Most people are reluctant to try new things until they reach a crisis, so why not add a few alternatives now before a crisis arises?

Recruit others to your favored activity and become an organizer and leader just for fun. Helping others enjoy your activity strengthens your own commitment to it as well. Share your passion with your spouse, friends, or co-workers and volunteer to help them get started. Eventually you'll build a personal support group that is dynamic and personally grateful to you. For example, you might start a neighborhood bicycling group on Saturday mornings, recruit others, plan interesting routes, and establish a reward system for those who participate regularly.

You might also consider recruiting your spouse or children to learn or try a new sport activity with you. Learning together adds an alternative activity for both of you, and you also get to the enjoy spending quality time together.

Another idea is to plan an exciting trip as a reward (e.g., an active golf, tennis, bicycling, skiing, or hiking vacation). Preparing physically for the trip will give you an incentive to be active, and the extrinsic reward of travel can be a strong motivational tool. Depending on your financial resources, such trips may be close to home or even feature travel and sightseeing in other countries.

Other options include taking some instruction to improve your skills, joining a competitive team, and competing in an event for your age group. With all this in mind, consider how you might spice up your current activity.

BUILDING YOUR OWN SUPPORT GROUP

If you aim for long-term success, it can be invaluable to surround yourself with people who support your behavior change, nutrition plan, and physical activity program. Such people can help you stay on track when life dishes up its distractions. And if they participate right along with you and reinforce your efforts, you'll enjoy facing the challenges together.

It may seem obvious, but the support of your immediate family members, with whom you interact every day, is often the most crucial. Your spouse, kids, or others living in your household can contribute daily to your success. From the time you begin implementing your program for change, you need to spend some time with family members, both individually and collectively, to help them understand exactly how they can support your effort. Don't be afraid to ask for their help. Do readily convey to them that you realize your new direction may at times inconvenience them.

As we mentioned in chapter 11, other people can be a source of strength, support, and motivation; they can also be saboteurs of your plan to become healthier and physically active. The people who are closest to you have the most influence and need to understand your commitment and motivations, and you should ask for their support. If they continually erect barriers for you by demanding your time for other things or emotionally withdraw their support, you may need to spend some time together communicating your individual needs and working toward a mutually agreeable compromise.

You can build a team of others who are on a similar path by joining groups, programs, or facilities. Joining with others engaged in similar pursuits helps you open lines of communication that allow you to share ideas, embrace challenges, and support solutions together. Just agreeing to meet regularly for physical activity with others takes your commitment to a new level, particularly if they can't do the activity (e.g., play tennis doubles) without you.

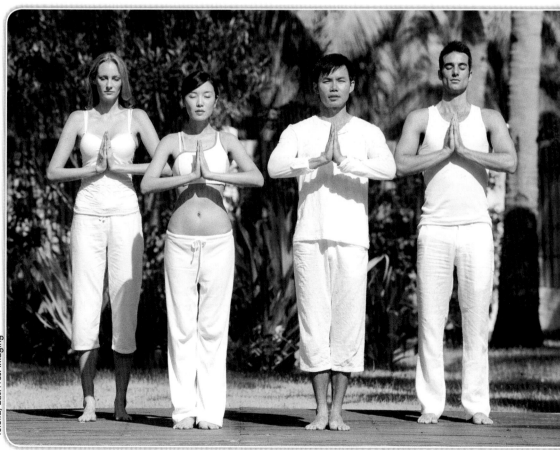

fotolia/EastWest Imaging

Group exercise solidifies your commitment to regular physical activity. If you don't show up, you'll be missed.

Beyond seeking support, you may also want to search for a mentor, someone who has more experience than you do and who is committed to goals for being physically active. This relationship may be just a friendly one or a professional one. If you are not paying for the service, look for ways in which you can compensate the person for advice with thoughtful gifts, invitations, or other services you can provide.

Be your own best friend throughout the process by being honest with yourself; accept hard truths when necessary. When you encounter challenges and difficulties, show patience and empathy. Think of your new commitment to healthy and physically active living as something that is in its infancy—and thus is alive and growing.

Rejoice when you see signs of growth and celebrate every success. Resist negative self-talk and disparaging remarks even when you mess up. Rather than obsessing about reaching specific goals, enjoy the journey to your new and higher level of personal energy.

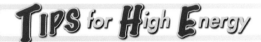

Tips for High Energy

- Learn to generate more personal energy through nutrition, rest and recovery, and physical activity.
- Manage your personal energy better by focusing your attention on investing your full and best energy here and now, in the present, rather than worrying about the past or the future.
- Strengthen your personal motivation by using intrinsic factors—based on your life's purpose and values as you see them—rather than relying solely on extrinsic rewards.
- Become your own coach for your energy quest by increasing your knowledge of the concepts, processes, and ritual building that are essential to achieving permanent changes in your behavior and lifestyle.
- Build an effective support group that can help you overcome barriers and provide ongoing emotional support as you establish new habits and rituals.

FITNESS TEST NORMS

Directions: Find your scores for the fitness tests in the following charts, which are arranged according to age and sex. Then enter your score in your personal test score result sheet (appendix 6).

Percentile rankings indicate the following rating:

90 = well above average
70 = above average
50 = average
30 = below average
10 = well below average

APPENDIX 1A	1-Minute Sit-Up Test (Men)				
	Age				
Percentile	**20-29**	**30-39**	**40-49**	**50-59**	**60+**
90	52	48	43	39	35
80	47	43	39	35	30
70	45	41	36	31	26
60	42	39	34	28	22
50	40	36	31	26	20
40	38	35	29	24	19
30	35	32	27	21	17
20	33	30	24	19	15
10	30	26	22	15	10

Data from *Physical Fitness Assessments and Norms for Adults and Law Enforcement.* Used with permission from The Cooper Institute, Dallas, Texas. For more information: www.cooperinstitute.org.

APPENDIX 1B 1-Minute Sit-Up Test (Women)

Percentile	Age				
	20-29	30-39	40-49	50-59	60+
90	49	40	34	29	26
80	44	35	29	24	17
70	41	32	27	22	12
60	38	29	24	20	11
50	35	27	22	17	8
40	32	25	20	14	6
30	30	22	17	12	4
20	24	20	14	10	3
10	21	15	10	6	1

Data from *Physical Fitness Assessments and Norms for Adults and Law Enforcement.* Used with permission from The Cooper Institute, Dallas, Texas. For more information: www.cooperinstitute.org.

APPENDIX 2A Push-Up Test (Men)

Percentile	Age				
	20-29	30-39	40-49	50-59	60-69
90	41	32	25	24	24
80	34	27	21	17	16
70	30	24	19	14	11
60	27	21	16	11	10
50	24	19	13	10	9
40	21	16	12	9	7
30	18	14	10	7	6
20	16	11	8	5	4
10	11	8	5	4	2

Source: *Canadian Standardized Test of Fitness Operations Manual, 3rd Edition,* Health Canada, 1986. Reproduced with permission of the Minister of Public Works and Government Services Canada, 2009.

APPENDIX 2B Push-Up Test (Women)

Percentile	Age				
	20-29	30-39	40-49	50-59	60-69
90	31	27	25	19	18
80	27	22	21	17	15
70	21	20	17	13	13
60	19	17	16	12	11
50	18	16	14	11	9
40	14	13	11	9	6
30	13	10	10	6	4
20	10	7	8	3	0
10	6	1	4	0	0

Reprinted, by permission, from V.H. Heyward, 2002, *Advanced fitness assessment and exercise prescription,* 4th ed. (Champaign, IL: Human Kinetics), 125. Data provided by the Women's Exercise Research Center, The George Washington University Medical Center, Washington, DC, 1998.

APPENDIX 3A Sit-and-Reach Test (Men)

Percentile	Age				
	20-29	30-39	40-49	50-59	60+
90	21.8	21.0	20.0	19.0	19.0
80	20.5	19.5	18.5	17.5	17.3
70	19.5	18.5	17.5	16.5	15.5
60	18.5	17.5	16.3	15.5	14.5
50	17.5	16.5	15.3	14.5	13.5
40	16.5	15.5	14.3	13.3	12.5
30	15.5	14.5	13.3	12.0	11.3
20	14.4	13.0	12.0	10.5	10.0
10	12.3	11.0	10.0	8.5	8.0

This table is based on using the "zero" point set at 15 inches (38 cm).

Data from *Physical Fitness Assessments and Norms for Adults and Law Enforcement.* Used with permission from The Cooper Institute, Dallas, Texas. For more information: www.cooperinstitute.org.

APPENDIX 3B Sit-and-Reach Test (Women)

	Age				
Percentile	**20-29**	**30-39**	**40-49**	**50-59**	**60+**
90	23.8	22.5	21.5	21.5	21.8
80	22.5	21.5	20.5	20.3	19.0
70	21.5	20.5	19.8	19.3	17.5
60	20.5	20.0	19.0	18.5	17.0
50	20.0	19.0	18.0	17.9	16.4
40	19.3	18.3	17.3	16.8	15.5
30	18.3	17.3	16.5	15.5	14.4
20	17.0	16.5	15.0	14.8	13.0
10	15.4	14.4	13.0	13.0	11.5

This table is based on using the "zero" point set at 15 inches (38 cm).

Data from *Physical Fitness Assessments and Norms for Adults and Law Enforcement.* Used with permission from The Cooper Institute, Dallas, Texas. For more information: www.cooperinstitute.org.

APPENDIX 4A 12-Minute Cooper Test (Men)

	Age					
Percentile	**20-29**	**30-39**	**40-49**	**50-59**	**60-69**	**70-79**
90	1.81	1.77	1.73	1.61	1.51	1.41
80	1.73	1.67	1.61	1.52	1.41	1.32
70	1.65	1.61	1.54	1.45	1.33	1.23
60	1.58	1.55	1.49	1.38	1.29	1.17
50	1.53	1.49	1.44	1.33	1.23	1.13
40	1.49	1.45	1.38	1.29	1.19	1.09
30	1.43	1.38	1.33	1.24	1.13	1.04
20	1.37	1.33	1.28	1.18	1.08	0.97
10	1.29	1.25	1.20	1.10	0.99	0.89

Note: distance covered in miles.

Data from *Physical Fitness Assessments and Norms for Adults and Law Enforcement.* Used with permission from The Cooper Institute, Dallas, Texas. For more information: www.cooperinstitute.org.

APPENDIX 4B   12-Minute Cooper Test (Women)

Percentile	Age					
	20-29	30-39	40-49	50-59	60-69	70-79
90	1.63	1.56	1.49	1.37	1.27	1.25
80	1.54	1.45	1.40	1.29	1.21	1.15
70	1.46	1.39	1.33	1.23	1.15	1.10
60	1.41	1.33	1.29	1.19	1.12	1.05
50	1.35	1.29	1.24	1.15	1.08	1.01
40	1.30	1.25	1.19	1.11	1.05	0.98
30	1.25	1.21	1.14	1.07	1.01	0.93
20	1.19	1.15	1.09	1.02	0.97	0.90
10	1.13	1.08	1.03	0.97	0.92	0.85

Note: distance covered in miles.

Data from *Physical Fitness Assessments and Norms for Adults and Law Enforcement.* Used with permission from The Cooper Institute, Dallas, Texas. For more information: www.cooperinstitute.org.

APPENDIX 5A   Percent Body Fat (Men)

Percentile	Age				
	20-29	30-39	40-49	50-59	60+
90	7.9	11.9	14.9	16.7	17.6
80	10.5	14.5	17.4	19.1	19.7
70	12.7	16.5	19.1	20.7	21.3
60	14.8	18.2	20.6	22.1	22.6
50	16.6	19.7	21.9	23.2	23.7
40	18.6	21.3	23.4	24.6	25.2
30	20.6	23.0	24.8	26.0	26.7
20	23.1	24.9	26.6	27.8	28.4
10	26.3	27.8	29.2	30.3	30.9

Data from *Physical Fitness Assessments and Norms for Adults and Law Enforcement.* Used with permission from The Cooper Institute, Dallas, Texas. For more information: www.cooperinstitute.org..

APPENDIX 5B   Percent Body Fat (Women)

Percentile	Age				
	20-29	30-39	40-49	50-59	60+
90	14.8	15.6	17.2	19.4	19.8
80	16.5	17.4	19.8	22.5	23.2
70	18.0	19.1	21.9	25.1	25.9
60	19.4	20.8	23.8	27.0	27.9
50	21.0	22.6	25.6	28.8	29.8
40	22.7	24.6	27.6	30.4	31.3
30	24.5	26.7	29.6	32.5	33.3
20	27.1	29.1	31.9	34.5	35.4
10	31.4	33.0	35.4	36.7	37.3

Data from *Physical Fitness Assessments and Norms for Adults and Law Enforcement.* Used with permission from The Cooper Institute, Dallas, Texas. For more information: www.cooperinstitute.org.

APPENDIX 6   My Fitness Results

Dates:

	Result	Result	Result	Result	Result
Cardiorespiratory (Cooper test)					
Muscular strength and endurance (push-up maximum)					
Muscular strength and endurance (sit-ups in 1 minute)					
Flexibility (sit-and-reach test)					
Body composition (percent body fat)					

From R. Woods and C. Jordan with the Human Performance Institute, 2010, *Energy every day* (Champaign, IL: Human Kinetics).

BIBLIOGRAPHY

American College of Sports Medicine. 1998. ACSM position stand: The recommended quantity and quality of exercise for developing and maintaining cardiorespiratory and muscular fitness, and flexibility in adults. *Medicine & Science in Sports & Exercise* 30 (6): 975–91.

American College of Sports Medicine. 2003. *ACSM fitness book: A proven step-by-step program from the experts.* 3rd ed. Champaign, IL: Human Kinetics.

American College of Sports Medicine. 2009. *Current Comments: Report on perceived exertion.* www.ascm.org/AM/Template.cfm?Section = current_comments1&templateCM/ ContentDisplay.cfm&ContentID8449 (accessed 5/23/2009).

Bargh, J.A., and T.L. Chartrand. 1999. The unbearable automaticity of being. *American Psychologist* 54 (7): 462–79.

Centers for Disease Control and Prevention. 2008. *How much physical activity do adults need?* www.cdc.gov/physicalactivity/everyone/guidelines/adults.html.

Top ten reasons to exercise. 2006. *Cherokee Sentinel,* January 11. www.cherokeesentinel. com/news/2006/0111/home/041.html.

Clark, N. 2008. *Nancy Clark's sports nutrition guidebook.* 4th ed. Champaign, IL: Human Kinetics.

Cooper, K. 1968. A means of assessing maximal oxygen uptake. *Journal of the American Medical Association* 203: 201–04.

Doidge, N. 2007. *The brain that changes itself.* New York: Penguin Books.

Groppel, J. 1997 *The anti-diet book.* Orlando: Human Performance Institute.

Harvard Health Publications with L. Epstein. 2008. *Improving sleep: A guide to a good night's rest.* Boston: Harvard Medical School.

Loehr, J. 2007. *The power of story.* New York: Free Press

National Cancer Institute. 2008. *Physical Activity and Cancer: Questions and Answers.* www. cancer.gov/cancertopics/factsheet/physical-activity-qa/print?page = &keyword = (accessed 5/18/2009).

National Center for Health Statistics. 2004. *Prevalence of overweight and obesity among adults: United States, 2003–2004.* www.cdc.gov/nchs/products/pubs/pubd/hestats/ overweight/overwght_adult_03.htm.

The President's Council on Physical Fitness and Sports. 1998. *Physical activity and aging: Implications for health and quality of life in older persons.* U.S. Department of Health and Human Services. www.fitness.gov/digest_dec1998.htm.

Ratey, J. 2008. *Spark.* New York: Little, Brown.

Simon, H. 2008. *Harvard Men's Health Watch,* September. www.health.harvard.edu/ healthbeat/HEALTHbeat_091608.htm.

Weinberg, R., and D. Gould. 2007. *Foundations of sport and exercise psychology.* Champaign, IL: Human Kinetics.

INDEX

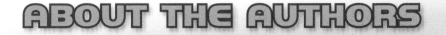

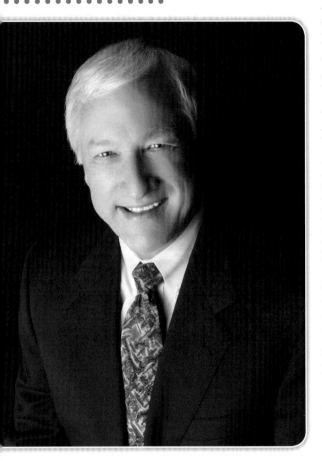

Ron Woods, PhD, is a performance coach for the Human Performance Institute (HPI) in Orlando, Florida, and an adjunct professor of sport science at the University of Tampa and the University of South Florida. He spent 20 years with the United States Tennis Association, including 10 years as the USTA's director of Player Development, a program that develops top junior players into touring professionals. For 17 years, Woods was professor of physical education and men's tennis coach at West Chester University. He has been inducted into West Chester University's Athletic Hall of Fame. A graduate of East Stroudsburg University and an inductee into their athletic hall of fame, Woods received his PhD from Temple University with an emphasis in sport psychology and motor learning. The International Tennis Hall of Fame awarded Ron the Educational Merit Award in 1997. He was also honored by the United States Professional Tennis Association (USPTA) as National Coach of the Year in 1982 and named a master professional in 1984. His accomplishments include eight years on the Coaching Committee of the United States Olympic Committee and the Coaches' Commission of the International Tennis Association. Woods authored *Social Issues in Sport* and *Playing Tennis After 50* and has written and edited numerous USTA publications, including *Coaching Youth Tennis, Tennis Tactics,* and *Coaching Tennis Successfully,* all published by Human Kinetics. He lives in St. Petersburg, Florida.

Chris Jordan is the vice president of facilitator training at HPI, the manager of its Corporate Athlete Train-the-Trainer course, and the director of fitness. Jordan manages the development and execution of all corporate fitness programs. He is also a regular contributor to *Men's Health, Best Life, Florida Tennis,* and *Outside* magazines. He holds a master of science degree in exercise physiology from Leeds Metropolitan University and a bachelor of science in applied biological sciences from the University of West England in Bristol. Before joining HPI, Jordan was the fitness program consultant for the U.S. Air Force in Europe at the Royal Air Force base in Lakenheath. He was also an exercise physiologist at the British Army Personnel Research Establishment of the Ministry of Defence. He is a certified strength and conditioning specialist and a certified personal trainer through the National Strength and Conditioning Association and a health fitness specialist and advanced personal trainer through the American College of Sports Medicine. Jordan lives in Orlando, Florida.

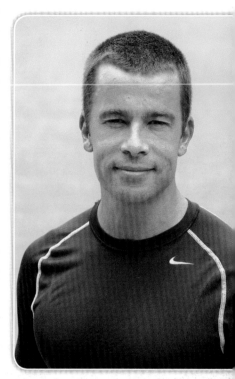

Headquartered in Orlando, Florida, the **Human Performance Institute** is the world leader in energy management technology. The institute's corporate athlete training solutions include executive and on-site training courses, keynotes, and Train-the-Trainer courses. Corporate clients include Procter & Gamble, the Estée Lauder companies, Dell, the FBI, GlaxoSmithKline, PepsiCo, and Morgan Stanley Smith Barney.

*You'll find
other outstanding
sports and fitness resources at*

www.HumanKinetics.com

In the U.S. call

1-800-747-4457

Australia.............................. 08 8372 0999
Canada 1-800-465-7301
Europe......................+44 (0) 113 255 5665
New Zealand.................. 0064 9 448 1207

HUMAN KINETICS
The Premier Publisher for Sports & Fitness
P.O. Box 5076 • Champaign, IL 61825-5076 USA